Psychosocial Nursing Care

Psychosocial Nursing Care

A Guide to Nursing
the Whole Person

Dave Roberts

McGraw Hill Education Open University Press

Open University Press
McGraw-Hill Education
McGraw-Hill House
Shoppenhangers Road
Maidenhead
Berkshire
England
SL6 2QL

email: enquiries@openup.co.uk
world wide web: www.openup.co.uk

and Two Penn Plaza, New York, NY 10121-2289, USA

First published 2013

A catalogue record of this book is available from the British Library

ISBN-13: 978-0-335-24414-0
ISBN-10: 0-335-24414-9
eISBN: 978-0-335-24415-7

Library of Congress Cataloging-in-Publication Data
CIP data applied for

Typeset by Aptara, Inc.

Fictitious names of companies, products, people, characters and/or data
that may be used herein (in case studies or in examples) are not intended
to represent any real individual, company, product or event.

Praise for this book

Dedication

For Farzaneh and Niayesh

Contents

Acknowledgements

I would like to thank a number of people who have made a particular contribution to the development of this book. My thanks go to the anonymous reviewers who helped to shape the book in its early stages. I am also particularly grateful to Rachel Crookes of Open University Press, who approached me about the book in the first place, and who made a number of very constructive and helpful suggestions at various stages of the writing and editing process.

I would like to thank Farzaneh Yazdani and Mark Foulkes who both provided very thoughtful feedback on several of the chapters, and Gail Eva, Peter Zaagman and Caral Stevenson who made a particular contribution on specific topics. I would also like to thank DIPEx for their kind permission to make extensive use of quotations from their interviews. There are many colleagues and patients I have worked with over the years whose experience, thoughts and ideas have had an influence on me and on my understanding of nursing. A big thank you to all of you.

And finally, thanks to Farzaneh and Niayesh, James and Mary, for their continual emotional support and for tolerating my absences.

Introduction

Psychosocial Nursing Care

Nursing should be care of the whole person, but anyone who has practised as a nurse knows that this can be very difficult to achieve. Day-to-day nursing is full of frustrations: interruptions and competing demands on time, bureaucracy, management structures, shortages of staff and resources can all make it difficult to provide holistic nursing care. Health care has become progressively more specialized, and most nursing activity has a very specific focus. Care may also be dictated by the patient's most urgent needs and the imperative to achieve effective resource management.

However, in addition to these wider, structural issues, nurses often lack the skills, knowledge and confidence to take on the care of the whole person. Opportunities are frequently missed to deal with psychological and social issues, as the nurse focuses on those areas that they know well and feel most comfortable dealing with. This problem is often attributed to the dominance of the medical model in health care, but it is possible to provide holistic care alongside medical treatments. The nurse simply needs to find their own voice in the system. This book aims to help the reader to develop the knowledge, skills and confidence to deal with the psychosocial aspects of care.

The patient's voice also needs to be heard. I have tried to give space to the patient's voice within this book. They know best what it feels like to be ill and to be on the receiving end of care and treatment. Patient-centred care means putting the patient's experience at the centre of the caring process, and this book explores how that voice can be heard, through patient narratives.

So, if there have been missed opportunities in the past, what can we do to address these possibilities in the present? Chapter 1 explores the barriers to our understanding of the health of the mind and body, the key to developing holistic nursing. It also discusses how we can understand personal experience of illness and reactions to being ill. Chapter 2 highlights the central place of communication in nursing care. This is the foundation on which nursing is built, and the stronger this foundation, the better the nursing care. The next chapter builds on this foundation, exploring the potential of the nurse–patient relationship, and for nursing to be a therapy in its own right. Nursing as therapy has dropped out of favour as increasing demands are made on nursing time and energies. However, therapeutic nursing is not an addition to nursing care, but is the heart and soul of nursing. It holds the promise of greater patient (and nurse) satisfaction with care, and this is explored in Chapter 3.

Nurses have a significant potential role in the detection of mental illness in the physically ill, and exploring the interface between mental and physical health. This can only be based on psychosocial assessment, the theme of Chapter 4. The overlap between nursing and psychotherapy has been discussed since the pioneering work of Hildegard Peplau. Chapter 5 reviews the increasing evidence of the potential for nurses to apply psychotherapeutic approaches within or in addition to the nursing care they provide.

As mental illnesses are common in the physically ill, the remaining chapters explore how their nursing care can be improved. Anxiety and depression, the most common mental illnesses, are discussed in depth in Chapters 6 and 7, exploring the potential for better, more patient-centred nursing care. Chapter 8 focuses on psychotic conditions. People with psychoses struggle to find a place within health care systems, but any claim to holistic or patient-centred care should include the care of people undergoing the extremes of human experience. The last chapter explores the care of patients who present particular difficulties to the nurse. This includes challenging behaviours, self-harm and suicidal behaviour, and the misuse of alcohol and drugs.

Two additional themes run through the book: the importance of narrative as a means of understanding patient experiences of health and illness, and the role of reflection in developing nursing practice. These themes emerge in some form in each chapter. Narrative as a concept has the potential to unlock patient stories, whether these are brief or more detailed accounts of personal experience. Reflection points invite the reader to reflect on either their own experience of practice, or on the case scenarios, with the purpose of learning and developing practice. I have summarized the main points of each chapter, and the nursing care of specific groups of patients, at regular intervals throughout the book. This is meant to aid learning, not to direct it. There are also additional readings and resources indicated for those who want to carry on studying the topic in greater depth.

This is a book written by a practising nurse (who is also an academic) for other nurses in practice. Its aim is to support the development of practice, and the individual nurse's confidence in practice. Nursing is the most rewarding of professions, though often challenging. I invite you to rise to the challenge of developing your practice within an integrative psychosocial model of nursing care.

Dave Roberts

1

MIND, BODY AND ILLNESS
In Search of the Whole Person

Learning outcomes

By the end of this chapter, you should be able to:

- explore the main theoretical models underlying the care and treatment of the mind and body;
- understand how individuals and families respond and adjust to illness;
- identify the factors influencing how patient distress and concerns are expressed and interpreted in health care settings;
- practise in a holistic way that recognizes individual interpretations and meanings of illness and distress.

Introduction

Nurses aim to care for the whole person, to provide holistic care. However, there are a number of challenges in achieving this. Contemporary health care is based on a model that splits the mind and body, and this is mirrored in the delivery of services. Developing an understanding of this mind–body split and its consequences for nurses and patients is therefore vitally important if the nurse is to provide holistic nursing care. In order to integrate care of the mind and body, it is also important for nurses to understand how people react to illness and its effects.

Mind and body in nursing

Health care splits the mind and body in terms of the organization and training of most health professions. Mental illness is managed by mental health nurses and psychiatrists, and physical illness by general adult nurses and a variety of medical specialists. In many ways this is a valid division of labour, and it has facilitated the high degree of specialization that we find in contemporary health care.

However, there are a number of problems that result from this mind–body split. First, psychological and physical health problems often exist side by side and are interrelated, so effective assessment and care can only be achieved by managing them both together. Chapters 6 and 7, for example, explore interrelationships between anxiety and depression and physical illness. Second, patients themselves may not experience this separation subjectively; for example, pain and anxiety may be a single unpleasant feeling. Patients develop their own personal understanding and *narrative* of illness, and this is explored in this chapter and Chapters 3 and 4. Third, our understanding of illness increasingly shows evidence of the interdependence between the physical and psychological aspects of health. Importantly, we now know that psychological treatments can have an impact on some physical health outcomes, including the use of mindfulness-based treatments in people with chronic pain and other long-term conditions (see Chapter 5).

This mind–body split has its roots within the philosophy of Descartes, which stated that mental and physical substance are essentially different and separate. This is referred to as Cartesian Dualism. Mental substance in this philosophical context can be seen to include both the mind and the spirit, existing within the inner conscious or unconscious world of the individual. Physical substance is essentially different in that it is observable and measurable in the outside world. There is undoubted value in this separation. The physical aspects of health, in terms of, for example, the properties of blood and tissue, and the effects of drug treatments, are amenable to observation and measurement. This is the basis of medical research into treatment effects, and of evidence-based practice, a fundamental aspect of contemporary health care. However, although the mind is more difficult to observe and measure, some aspects of mental life are observable and measurable. Thoughts and feelings can be observed or reported, and it is possible to undertake measurements of mood and other aspects of mental behaviour. Within the science of neurology, it is possible to make very explicit links between mental behaviour and physical changes in the nervous system, and the science of psychoneuroimmunology has established links between mental state and physical health, providing a model for understanding autoimmune diseases.

Within nursing, there has been a reaction against Cartesian Dualism as being inconsistent with caring values and the realities and complexities of nursing practice. Many nursing theorists reject the mind–body split in favour of a view of the person (both patient and nurse) as having a consciousness that is embodied (experienced within a body) and is part of a world where their experiences and actions have significance and meaning (Lepper 1998). These different views – a broader view of the whole person within context, and a more narrow view that reduces people to their constituent parts in order to study and understand them – can be described as holism and reductionism (see Box 1.1).

Box 1.1 Mind, body and nursing: key terminology

- **Dualism**, or **Cartesian Dualism**   A philosophical position stating that mind and body are separate and have a different nature or substance.
- **Holism**   The idea that any system, for example people, families, should be viewed as a whole. This whole system cannot be understood solely in terms of its component parts; that is, the whole is greater than the sum of its parts.

- **Reductionism** In contrast to holism, reductionism states that phenomena are best understood by reduction to their constituent parts.
- **Integration** An approach to knowledge that combines elements of different perspectives or different disciplines to achieve a synthesis.
- **Existential** Universal and fundamental concerns about the purpose and meaning of life. These become prominent at times when life and health are threatened.

Holism, reductionism

Nurses aim to care for the whole person, and many would claim a commitment to the principles of holism. Put simply, holism views people as more than the sum of their parts. This is in contrast to the way that people are often treated in health care organizations, which separate them into their different biological and psychological systems for the purpose of diagnosis and treatment. In practice an emphasis on holistic approaches in nursing means looking beyond the immediate diagnostic and treatment condition of the patient to a broader view of their needs. This includes spiritual aspects of both the nurse's and patient's experience. *Holistic nursing* is a term that focuses nursing on the whole person, including their unique experience of health and illness, promoting nursing as a healing agent, incorporating complementary therapies and self-awareness in the nurse (American Holistic Nurses Association 2012).

Nursing theorists have argued that holism offers a philosophical medium for expressing the complexity of nursing practice, and for nursing the whole person, within their social and environmental context. It provides an alternative to the reductionist approach to the person, represented by medicine and medical research, which reduces the person to physiological and psychological symptoms and systems (Risjord 2010). However, in spite of its many attractions in terms of validating and explaining the nurses' perspective, holism presents a number of problems.

First, seeing the sum of the whole as greater than the parts begs the question, *'what is the whole?'* – the patient, the family, the health care system or society? Second, the 'reductionist' medical system has many benefits to both patient and nurse in terms of constantly improving treatments. If holism is to have value to nurses in practice, then it has to be flexible enough to identify different units of care (or 'wholes') under different circumstances, and it has to find an accommodation with conventional science, bearing in mind that not all doctors or medical scientists would identify themselves as reductionists anyway.

One resolution of this dilemma is to recognize that holism as a philosophy can have subtle distinctions. Pragmatic holism (Woods 1998) or practical holism (Risjord 2009) allow its scope to be adjusted according to the context. While all aspects of the patient's health require attention, each may be considered separately. For example, in the case of pain, the following could be considered in planning nursing care:

- the patient's nervous system as the medium for analgesic treatment;
- their psychological state, anxiety;
- the social context, their interaction with family members and health care staff, which can impact on how they experience the pain;

- their experience of *total pain*, which may be considered to have a spiritual dimension;
- the health system within which their care takes place and the adequacy of resources to meet their needs.

Holism is, therefore, a suitable philosophical basis for nursing, if it is used in a flexible and pragmatic way.

Integration

Nurses face other challenges in caring for the whole person. In the main, general adult nurses are employed to look after sick bodies and this is what society expects them to do (Lawler 1991). With global restrictions on resources, money is allocated to deal with specific health problems, and this is true of both centrally funded systems like the British National Health Service, and other largely insurance-funded systems in other parts of the world. Nurses are therefore under pressure to focus their care on the patient's main presenting problem.

Under these circumstances, it can be particularly difficult to nurse the whole person. Nurses will need to make a case for the care they provide based on its health-related outcomes, effectiveness, and at times its cost-effectiveness. The nurse's ally in this is likely to be the patient. Patients and their families want to receive effective nursing care. In addition, patients want their voice to be heard, their experience of illness, and their personal narrative to be understood. The nurse is very well positioned, because of their proximity to the patient, and because of their focus on the relationship with the patient, to hear this voice.

Effective care is therefore not only evidence-based, but also takes a holistic view of the patient's needs, and incorporates the patient's own narrative of their illness and treatment. The nurse needs to focus on their relationship with the patient as a person in order to achieve this. This book therefore presents an *integrated approach to nursing care*, integrating physical, psychological, social and spiritual elements of the patient's experience and condition, in both assessment and care planning (see Boxes 1.2 and 1.3).

Box 1.2 Mind and spirit

Many of our words for aspects of the mind, for example, *psychological, psychiatric*, derive from a Greek word, ψυχή *(psyche)*, which means soul. Descartes' original thoughts on Dualism envisioned the mind and the soul as essentially the same. Psyche also has the meaning in English of the whole mind, including those aspects of the mind that are intangible and unobservable. There is a real sense, then, that the mind has hidden depths that cannot be readily studied or measured, but that are a significant part of human experience. We can make a distinction between psychological and spiritual aspects of human experience, though in practice, particularly in terms of personal meaning in life, they may be describing the same thing.

Speck et al (2004) identify that a number of different terms are used to describe aspects of spirituality within the context of health care. These refer to the life and death, or *existential*, issues that face us all, particularly when ill, and how we respond to them through processes of *coping, connecting, becoming*, and *finding value and meaning* in our life and world. This often involves a re-evaluation of personal identity. Some people also seek dimensions of s*piritual* experience beyond the self, sometimes termed *transcendence*. While many people do find this through *religion*, for others a more *philosophical* approach describes their search for meaning without the need to identify a spiritual power outside of the self. There has been a tendency to assume that spirituality and religion mean the same thing. However, it is increasingly recognized that not all spiritual needs are met by religion.

Within this book, the mental life of the individual is primarily referred to in terms of psychological aspects of experience and needs. This may include the spirit, but this is interpreted as an essentially more personal, and less tangible, aspect of the mind. Spirituality is often a distinctly personal experience, and some people would not use this term at all to describe their mental life. Each individual needs to find personal meaning in their experience of life and illness, and to find sources of strength within themselves, their family, friends and community, and in external ideas or power they perceive as greater than themselves.

Box 1.3 Psyche and soma

The term *soma,* referring to the body, is, like *psyche*, from the Greek. The term *somatic symptom*, for example, is used to describe a physical symptom in contrast to a psychological one. Psychosomatic as a term has had a number of meanings in health care. *Psychosomatic medicine* came to be associated in the early twentieth century with a movement towards a less reductionist, more integrative approach to the study and treatment of illness. By the 1950s, the term *psychosomatic disorders* was used to describe a causative relationship between psychological states and certain physical illnesses, including duodenal ulcer, ulcerative colitis and rheumatoid arthritis (Lipowski 1982). More recent research suggests more complex relationships between physical and psychological states where causation is often unclear.

The concept of psychosomatic disorder is now generally not used, but 'psychosomatic' remains in use in psychosomatic medicine and *psychosomatic research*. Psychosomatic research refers to the study of interrelationships between physical and mental health. Psychosomatic medicine has become synonymous with *liaison psychiatry*, which is the branch of psychiatry dealing with the overlap between mental and physical health, often based in the general hospital. A branch of mental health nursing, *mental health liaison nursing*, similarly addresses areas of coexisting psychological and physical health problems (Roberts 1997).

How people react to illness

In working with people going through the changes associated with illness, it is intriguing and sometimes surprising to see how people react differently to similar circumstances. There are a number of factors that determine an individual person's response to illness. These include:

- previous experience of illness in self and others;
- interpretations of the meaning and significance of illness events (including health beliefs);
- available information, knowledge and cultural assumptions about illness;
- personal appraisal of own ability to deal effectively with current demands and to remain in control of events (ability to cope);
- level of professional and social support available.

There are also different models that we can use to understand individual reactions and how we can respond to them in the most helpful way for the patient and their family.

Stress, coping and adjustment

Coping is a well-established term to describe how people deal with the demands made on them, or *stress*, by how they think about them and how they respond to them. The way that we cope is strongly influenced by our *appraisal* of these demands. Appraisal means how we interpret the significance of an event for our lives, and how we evaluate our options and potential for coping (Lazarus and Folkman 1984). In the face of illness, for example, we may respond by seeing the illness as a threat or a challenge, and we could feel either that it is overwhelming and we are unable to cope, or that we can overcome it with the support of friends and family.

Coping can be characterized as:

- problem-focused coping (efforts to manage the problem)
- emotion-focused coping (efforts taken to regulate distress)
- meaning-based coping (efforts to maintain well-being)

(Folkman and Greer 2000)

Appraisal influences which form of coping is used. An appraisal of greater control in response to stress is likely to lead to problem-focused coping, for example seeking information and practical solutions, and will lead to more effective problem-solving. Problem-solving enhances personal control and reduces distress, and is a key factor in managing depression (see Chapter 7 – Working with the depressed person). An appraisal of less control is more likely to lead to emotion-focused coping. This has the potential to be less effective, for example, by seeking comfort and avoiding distress at the cost of not dealing with the problems. Meaning-based coping can come into play when events are difficult and unsatisfactory and a reappraisal takes place, often involving revision of personal goals and looking for meaning in changing circumstances (Folkman and Greer 2000).

   People usually have a characteristic coping style, which may involve dealing with problems, confiding and discussing problems with friends or family, or avoiding them through escape or alcohol misuse. At times of stress and personal crisis, it can be useful to review this, asking, what has helped me to cope in the past, and what have I done that has been unhelpful? Effective coping leads to a positive process of adjustment to illness.

Implications for nursing practice

In supporting patients through periods of illness and change, it is helpful to:

- review the patient's usual coping style and how effective it has been in the past and is now;
- identify current priorities and establish meaningful and realistic goals, encouraging behaviour towards achieving these goals;
- emphasize opportunities for personal control and problem-solving.

Case study: stress, coping and adjustment

Tracey Brown is 22 years old and has suffered leg fractures in a road traffic accident. She is finding it difficult to cope with the resulting restrictions on her activity. Previously, she visited the gym three or four times a week. She now feels bored, restless and frustrated, feels she has lost control of her life, and that she will not be able to get through the next few weeks. She had led a very busy life revolving around her job in customer service, the gym and her social life. At a fracture clinic attendance, she is talking to the nurse when she starts crying and says that she can't cope any more. In discussion with the nurse, it is clear that her high levels of activity helped her to deal with stress, and she just can't do this at the moment. The nurse asks if she has had problems in the past and how she dealt with them. Tracey says she has always kept busy as a way of coping. She explores alternative ways of keeping busy with the nurse, and decides to enrol on an online course that will help her career. This gives her a sense that there is something that she can do within her current limitations to keep in touch with her work and develop her future career, and this enables her to feel more in control of her life. This case is explored in more detail in Chapter 4 – Psychosocial assessment.

Transition and growth

Another way to understand reaction to illness is as a *psychosocial transition*. This means that difficult events can lead to both negative and positive outcomes, having the overall effect of triggering positive psychosocial change. This effect was first identified in the study of bereavement reactions, and has also been applied in adjustment to a diagnosis of cancer (Andrykowski et al 1993). The transition serves as a period of reflection and restructuring of the person's view of the world, alongside whatever negative effects the illness has. This could include, for example, developing an enhanced sense of personal values at the same time as a loss of physical function.

Brennan's (2001) *social cognitive transition model of adjustment* draws on this model and develops it by emphasizing the cognitive elements, how our assumptions about the world are confirmed or modified in response to demands, and how the social context impacts on this. Brennan emphasizes the *normal* elements of response to illness and seeks to identify where these may become maladaptive. For example, worry can be a way of mentally preparing for a 'worst case scenario', reflecting on the capacity to deal with a future threat. It becomes maladaptive when it fails to resolve the uncertainty posed by the threat. This model is consistent with *cognitive therapy*, which emphasizes belief structures and assumptions about the world as a focus for therapeutic change (see Chapter 5).

In seeking to *normalize* reactions to illness, Brennan (2001) identifies that shocking events or news may temporarily overwhelm an individual's capacity to make sense of the world, leading to a state of confusion and disorientation. Given that most people's assumptions about the world are flexible, this usually only lasts a few hours or days, as their assumptions are adapted to fit the new situation. This is a way of understanding *acute stress reactions or disorders*. People who hold more rigid assumptions about the world and have less capacity to adapt to them may be more prone to longer-lasting effects of stress, *post-traumatic stress disorder (PTSD)* (see Chapter 6 for a review of stress reactions and disorders).

However, reactions to trauma are not always negative or pathological. *Post-traumatic growth* (PTG) is a phenomenon where people not only overcome trauma but achieve a better level of functioning than before. This represents a positive response to adversity. PTG has been described in response to accidents and disasters and also to a range of conditions, including malignant disease, human immunodeficiency virus, renal dialysis, multiple sclerosis, diabetes mellitus, rheumatoid arthritis, myocardial infarction and cerebrovascular accident. A review of the literature on PTG identified several themes in people's lives associated with growth after trauma: reappraisal of life and personal priorities, finding new meaning in life and a sense of personal transformation. In addition, people with physical illness reported a changed relationship with their body that could lead to a greater sense of personal control and better awareness of health issues (Hefferon et al 2009).

Implications for nursing practice

- Assumptions about ourselves, others and the world may be challenged by significant events like accidents and illness: positive adaptation and adjustment depends on our capacity to adapt these assumptions to the new circumstances.

- Events in illness and treatment have inherent personal meaning for the patient and there is always the potential for them to find personal growth and development in the face of adversity.

- Opportunities for personal reflection, including writing, sharing thoughts and feelings and seeking support should be encouraged.

Case study: transition and growth

Gemma Turner is a 36-year-old woman with a recent diagnosis of breast cancer. Her immediate reaction has been one of fear and a conviction that she is going to die. Her own mother died of breast cancer when Gemma was a child and this has led her to take a very pessimistic view of cancer and its treatment. However, she has been told that her prognosis is good, and she is currently having active chemotherapy treatment. Gemma gets on very well with her breast care specialist nurse, who has been trained in some cognitive therapy techniques. The breast care nurse suggests that Gemma keeps a diary of positive events that occur during her treatment and what they mean for her life [an excerpt from Gemma's diary is given in Chapter 5, Figure 5.2, p. 87]. They review this together when she attends the clinic. The breast care nurse helps Gemma to focus on her positive experiences and to review the evidence for her prognosis. Gemma finds that many good things have come out of her illness, including more supportive relationships with friends and family, and she feels she can take positive steps to overcome the cancer. Several months later, after successfully ending treatment, she feels she is stronger than before the cancer, and feels that her own cancer story will be different from her mother's.

Resilience

Resilience is another way of understanding human reactions that has gained some popularity in health care circles. It is '…a dynamic process encompassing positive adaptation within the context of significant adversity' (Luthar et al 2000: 543). It is therefore similar to transition and post-traumatic growth models. For resilience to be present, there are two conditions:

- exposure to significant threat or adversity;
- achievement of positive adaptation.

Unlike coping, resilience represents a focus on strengths rather than problems, though both protective factors and vulnerability can be identified in individuals. Resilience has the distinct quality of positive adaptation when the expectation would be that a 'normal' response would be less adaptive (Luthar et al 2000). Resilience may be identified within individuals, families or communities, and a resilient individual is likely to have personal strengths, a supportive family and to live in a community that provides adequate support. In terms of personality, it is associated with:

- self-esteem
- assertiveness
- hardiness
- flexibility

- energy
- humour
- a capacity for regulating emotions

(Agaibi and Wilson 2005)

Resilience is also associated with internal *locus of control*, that is, a sense that the person believes they can control their life, in contrast to external locus of control, where the person believes that their life is primarily controlled by outside factors.

Within a family context, resilience can be seen as maintaining core functions of the family:

- cohesion, membership, identity
- economic support
- nurturance, education, socialization
- protection of vulnerable members

(Zaider and Kissane 2007)

Implications for nursing practice

- Individuals, families and communities may have intrinsic resilience or vulnerability: resources should be targeted on providing support for those who have least resilience.
- Nurses should promote resilience through self-efficacy and personal control in patients and families.

Case study: resilience

Andy Clarke is 65 and has been diagnosed with diabetes. He lives alone but has three adult children who see him regularly. He has been having difficulty adjusting to the changes that are necessary in his lifestyle due to the illness. This has included changes to his diet, and he has found this particularly difficult as he has always eaten a carbohydrate-rich diet based on the foods from his country of origin, Jamaica. He feels that his diet is part of his identity and he is very reluctant to give it up. The staff at his local health centre are concerned about how he will cope and what effects non-compliance would have on his health. However, his children help him to try out new recipes and combinations of foods that suit his taste. He also finds a lot of strength from his church, whose members have helped him with regular support and adapted to changes, for example, when they share meals together. He manages to change his diet and adapt to his condition with his sense of personal and cultural identity intact. Andy says he has had a hard life but has survived through the support of his family, his church and his community. This case is explored further in Chapter 4 – Psychosocial assessment.

Psychopathology and comorbidity

As well as the range of reactions identified so far, people with physical illness also experience mental health problems. Within psychiatry, evidence of mental health problems is identified in signs and symptoms found in personal experience and behaviour. These are organized under the term 'psychopathology', and diagnosis is based on the nature, duration, severity or effects of a symptom.

In terms of personal reactions to illness, potential psychiatric diagnoses are the acute stress reactions and disorders, PTSD, and *adjustment disorder*, which usually features the symptoms of anxiety and/or depression and is associated with an ongoing stressful situation. Within the context of physical illness, there are a number of other mental health problems that can be encountered in general nursing practice. These include:

- physical illness that presents as psychological disturbance (e.g. delirium, porphyria);
- psychological disturbance that presents as physical illness (e.g. somatization disorder);
- psychological disturbance associated with treatment (e.g. PTSD following a period in intensive care);
- physical illness that is associated with psychological disturbance (e.g. chronic pain and depression);
- comorbidity, where both physical and psychological conditions exist together (e.g. chronic heart disease and depression).

Psychological comorbidity is very common in the physically ill, most commonly depression. Around 20 per cent of people with long-term conditions have depression, and this is associated with poorer quality of life (Moussavi et al 2007). Depression and anxiety are the most common mental disorders in the general population. Patients who have anxiety or depression and a long-term medical condition report significantly higher numbers of physical symptoms than those with a long-term condition alone, and this is true across hospital and community settings (Katon et al 2007; Gili et al 2010). This comorbidity is associated with greater disability and use of health services (Escobar et al 2010).

Comorbidity between mental and physical disorders has considerable implications for patient experience and service provision. Generally, quality of life is worse when these conditions occur together than in either condition alone, and the use of services, and costs of service use are higher. The nature of the biological and psychosocial processes and causation underlying comorbidity is not clear, but it is likely that the following factors are involved:

- Anxiety and depression are associated with poor concordance with treatment, poor self-care and increased complications of disease.
- Anxiety and depression both lead to enhanced awareness of physical symptoms, and can cause some additional symptoms through muscular tension and autonomic nervous system arousal.

- Increased reporting of physical symptoms in patients with comorbid anxiety and depression leads to more medical tests and medication changes.
- Symptom experience and burden, and functional impairment, contribute to the development and maintenance of anxiety and depression.

(Katon et al 2007)

Medicalization and normalization

It is important, then, to understand when to support a 'normal' reaction to illness, and when we need to intervene to manage a distressing and treatable psychological state. Patients themselves may ask the nurse if their reactions or feelings are normal. There are different ways to think about answering this question. Abnormal can have the meaning of pathological, that is, an abnormal psychological reaction. The key consideration is whether the patient has a treatable mental condition. However, there has been considerable debate about whether human reactions to illness should be *medicalized*, that is, treated as an illness. The alternative to this is *normalization*, understanding the person's reaction as a normal response to the circumstances.

For example, a patient experiencing the shock of a diagnosis of serious illness may react by crying all the time. For some people, this would be very shocking, as they do not consider this to be normal for them. However, we know that crying is a normal expression of distress. It could be helpful then for the nurse to normalize the patient's experience by reassuring them that they would consider tearfulness to be normal or understandable under these circumstances. On the other hand, persistent tearfulness over an extended period of time, accompanied by other features such as loss of pleasure and enjoyment of life, feelings of low mood and worthlessness, can be a feature of depression. Depression is a treatable condition (see Chapter 7). So, it is helpful to the patient to identify the nature of the problem that they are experiencing, and to discuss with them the options for managing the depression. Rather than medicalize the problem, in the sense of making their experience abnormal, this can have the effect of empowering them by giving their sense of distress a name and also a means to overcome it (Salmon et al 1999).

Medically unexplained physical symptoms and somatoform disorders

The debate becomes more complex when we look at *medically unexplained physical symptoms (MUPS)*. These are presentations of physical symptoms for which no explanation can be found using standard medical tests. They are associated with frequent presentations in primary care and extensive investigations. MUPS are usually understood as an expression of the psychological or social state of the patient, rather than representing a physical illness. Patients who have medically unexplained symptoms may feel that they are not taken seriously or that they are being told 'it is all in your mind'.

The process by which these symptoms develop is often described in terms of the patient's *attributional style*. Examples are: *normalizing* symptoms such as fatigue 'I am tired because I have been working hard', *somatizing* 'I am tired because I have had a virus and I am ill', or *psychologizing* 'I am tired because I am depressed' (Burton 2003). These personal styles may demonstrate a consistent pattern whatever the cause of the symptoms, and sometimes attributions are maintained in the face of contrary evidence, that is, medical tests that demonstrate an absence of pathology. However, in some cases they are amenable to change by psychotherapy (Morriss et al 1999; Dowrick et al 2004).

MUPS constitute a high proportion of presentations in primary care, and can include various pains: headaches, facial pain, non-cardiac chest pain, pelvic pain, fibromyalgia and also fatigue. MUPS do not usually present as single symptoms, and frequently include a number of symptoms together. They are often associated with psychological problems like anxiety and depression, and this is more likely when there is a higher number of symptoms (Burton 2003).

Psychiatry usually interprets MUPS as a form of somatization, that is, the attribution by the patient of a physical cause to the reported problem. This is different from somatization disorder, which is a discrete syndrome with very specific diagnostic criteria (Mai 2004). There is a range of unresolved physical problems that are thought to have psychological origins, falling under the general diagnostic category of somatoform disorders (see Box 1.4).

Box 1.4 Somatoform disorders (according to DSM-IV classification)

- *Conversion disorder*, where the symptoms have the appearance of neurological disorder, but there is no underlying neurological cause.
- *Hypochondriasis,* also called Health Anxiety, an excessive preoccupation with having a serious physical illness (see Chapter 6).
- *Body dysmorphic disorder*, an excessive concern with body image, focusing on a perceived physical defect.
- *Pain disorder*, severe disabling and sometimes long-lasting pain that is in excess of the original cause.
- *Somatization disorder*, recurring, multiple, clinically significant complaints about pain, gastrointestinal, sexual and pseudoneurological symptoms.

Psychotherapeutic approaches to managing MUPS aim either to *reattribute* the cause of the symptoms to a psychosocial one, or to explore reasons for the MUPS in a way that *normalizes* them (Box 1.5). Both of these models have been taught to doctors in primary care, with good outcomes in terms of the patient's mental state and function (Morriss et al 1999; Dowrick et al 2004).

However, in spite of evidence that these psychotherapeutic approaches are of benefit to patients who somatize, there are voices that are critical of the idea that the problem lies solely with the patient. One criticism is that the dualistic nature of medicine leads to a psychological cause being sought if no physical cause is found. This excludes social and cultural factors that may provide a credible explanation for

---

Box 1.5 Medically unexplained physical symptoms: reattribution and normalization

Reattribution:
(a) Demonstrating understanding of the patient's condition.
(b) Reframing the problem, through negotiation, in terms of the psychological information provided by the patient.
(c) Making links between distress and reported symptoms using explanatory models.

(Morriss et al 1999)

Normalization:
(a) Listening and acknowledging the patient's suffering.
(b) Providing explanations for the symptoms causing concern.
(c) Exploring links between psychological factors and physical mechanisms.

(Dowrick et al 2004)

---

the somatic presentation of psychological and social problems. Mental illness attracts stigma whereas physical illness generally does not, so MUPS may represent a socially acceptable expression of distress. Kirmayer et al (2004) suggest that many cultures have *sociosomatic* explanations of the distress that arises from family and community problems, so somatization is a common culturally sanctioned process. The health care setting, then, needs to provide opportunities for distress to be explored through the patient's own narrative, to discover inherent personal and cultural meanings.

Case study: medically unexplained physical symptoms

Mrs Lakshmi Patel is a 32-year-old married woman with three young children. She has been attending her local health centre regularly over the last three months complaining of aches and pains in various parts of her body. She has been examined by the GP on a number of occasions and had various tests that have not identified anything abnormal. The practice nurse sees her for a routine appointment and has the time to ask her more about how she is feeling. Mrs Patel seems reluctant to discuss her life with the practice nurse, who feels she may have concerns about confidentiality. She reassures her that their conversation is private and confidential. Mrs Patel implies that she has some concerns about her marriage and does not feel close to her husband at the moment, but she does not want to go into detail. The practice nurse suggests a referral to the practice counsellor but Mrs Patel is also reluctant to talk to her. The practice nurse identifies some features of depression, including sleep and appetite disturbance (she is comfort eating and has put on weight) and a general sense of dissatisfaction with life. She asks Mrs Patel if she would consider taking antidepressant medication, which Mrs Patel says she will consider if it will help with her aches and pains. Mrs Patel agrees to see the GP to discuss this (see Chapter 5 for a further discussion of this case).

Reflection point

Do you think this would be a satisfactory outcome from Mrs Patel's point of view? Is there anything else you could suggest that might help her to deal with her problems?

There are other problems that have been identified through qualitative analysis of interviews between general practitioners (GPs) and patients. Contrary to the belief that patients only present physical symptoms, and seek physical explanations and medical tests, this study found that patients frequently provided *cues* (see Chapter 3) to their psychosocial concerns. This included statements about uncertainty, social and domestic problems, stress and mood. However, it was the doctors who frequently kept the focus on somatic complaints and investigations, sometimes disregarding cues of a more emotional character (Salmon et al 2004). The success of reattribution therapy may be because it focuses the doctor's attention on these psychosocial cues. There is therefore a compelling case for framing the problem of MUPS and somatization within the professional–patient interaction (Goldberg and Bridges 1988).

Summary

This chapter has discussed the nature of holism, the nature of personal reactions to illness, and other concepts that are relevant to nursing practice. It has also begun to explore how interaction is central to the nurse–patient relationship, and how nurses can effectively support patients who are going through difficult periods of adjustment and transition as a result of illness. The next chapter – Communication in nursing – explores some of the practical ways that nurses can engage with the patient and manage the health-related problems that they encounter.

Key points

- Practical or pragmatic holism is a suitable theoretical basis for psychosocial nursing practice.
- Personal reactions to illness have the potential for personal growth as well as leading to personal problems.
- Psychological problems associated with physical illness include relatively straightforward conditions like anxiety and depression, and less common, more complex conditions like somatization and MUPS.
- Psychotherapy may help people with somatoform disorders, whether the cause of the illness is physical or psychosocial.
- A holistic approach to the presentation of symptoms and concerns is more likely to uncover personal and cultural meaning inherent in the symptom experience, and facilitate the expression of patient concerns in the patient's own terms.

References

Agaibi, C.E. and Wilson, J.P. (2005) Trauma, PTSD, and resilience, *Trauma, Violence & Abuse*, 6 (3), 195–216.

American Holistic Nurses Association (2012) Available online at www.ahna.org/AboutUs/WhatisHolisticNursing/tabid/1165/Default.aspx

Andrykowski, M., Brady, M. and Hunt, J. (1993) Positive psychosocial adjustment in potential bone marrow transplant recipients: cancer as a psychosocial transition, *Psycho-oncology*, 2, 261–276.

Brennan, J. (2001) Adjustment to cancer – coping or personal transition? *Psycho-oncology*, 10 (1), 1–18.

Burton, C. (2003) Beyond somatisation: a review of the understanding and treatment of medically unexplained physical symptoms (MUPS), *British Journal of General Practice*, 53, 233–241.

Dowrick, C., Ring, A., Humphris, G. and Salmon, P. (2004) Normalisation of unexplained symptoms by general practitioners: a functional typology, *British Journal of General Practice*, 54, 165–170.

Escobar, J., Cook, B., Chen, C-N., Gara, M., Alegria, M., Interian, A. and Diaz, E. (2010) Whether medically explained or not, three or more concurrent somatic symptoms predict psychopathology and service use in community populations, *Journal of Psychosomatic Research*, 69, 1–8.

Folkman, S. and Greer, S. (2000) Promoting psychological well-being in the face of serious illness: when theory, research and practice inform each other, *Psycho-oncology*, 9, 11–19.

Gili, M., Comas, A., Garcia-Garcia, M., Monzon, S., Serrano-Blanco, A. and Roca, M. (2010) Comorbidity between common mental disorders and chronic somatic diseases in primary care patients, *General Hospital Psychiatry*, 32, 240–245.

Goldberg, D. and Bridges, K. (1988) Somatic presentations of psychiatric illness in primary care setting, *Journal of Psychosomatic Research*, 32 (2), 137–144.

Hefferon, K., Grealy, M. and Mutrie, N. (2009) Post-traumatic growth and life threatening physical illness: a systematic review of the qualitative literature, *British Journal of Health Psychology*, 14, 343–378.

Katon, W., Lin, E. and Kroenke, K. (2007) The association of depression and anxiety with medical symptom burden in patients with chronic medical illness, *General Hospital Psychiatry*, 29, 147–155.

Kirmayer, L., Groleau, D., Looper, K. and Dao, M. (2004) Explaining medically unexplained symptoms, *Canadian Journal of Psychiatry*, 49 (10), 663–672.

Lawler, J. (1991) *Behind the Screens: Nursing, Somology, and the Problem of the Body*. Melbourne: Churchill Livingstone.

Lazarus, R.S. and Folkman, S. (1984) *Stress, Appraisal, and Coping*. New York: Springer Publishing Company.

Lepper, E. (1998) Towards a credible theory of mind for nursing, in Edwards, S. (ed.) *Philosophical Issues in Nursing*. Basingstoke: Macmillan, pp. 109–125.

Lipowski, Z.J. (1982) Modern meaning of the terms 'psychosomatic' and 'liaison psychiatry', in Creed, F. and Pfeffer, J.M. (eds) *Medicine and Psychiatry: A Practical Approach*. London: Pitman, pp. 3–24.

Luthar, S., Cicchetti, D. and Becker, B. (2000) The construct of resilience: a critical evaluation and guidelines for future work, *Child Development*, 71 (3), 543–562.

Mai, F. (2004) Somatization disorder: a practical review, *Canadian Journal of Psychiatry*, 49 (10), 652–662.

Morriss, R., Gask, L., Ronalds, C., Downes-Grainger, E., Thompson, H. and Goldberg, D. (1999) Clinical and patient satisfaction outcomes of a new treatment for somatised mental disorder taught to general practitioners, *British Journal of General Practice*, 49, 263–267.

Moussavi, S., Chatterji, S., Verdes, E., Tandon, A., Patel, V. and Ustun, B. (2007) Depression, chronic diseases, and decrements in health: results from the World Health Surveys, *The Lancet*, 370 (9590), 808–809.

Risjord M. (2009) Reductionism and holism. Available online at www.nursingknowledge. wordpress.com/category/holism-and-reductionism/

Risjord M. (2010) *Nursing Knowledge. Science, Practice, and Philosophy*. Chichester: Wiley Blackwell.

Roberts, D. (1997) Liaison mental health nursing: origins, definition and prospects, *Journal of Advanced Nursing*, 25 (1), 101–108.

Salmon, P., Peters, S. and Stanley, I. (1999) Patients' perceptions of medical explanations for somatisation disorders: qualitative analysis, *British Medical Journal*, 318, 372–376.

Salmon, P., Dowrick, C., Ring, A. and Humphris, G. (2004) Voiced but unheard agendas: qualitative analysis of the psychosocial cues that patients with unexplained symptoms present to general practitioners, *British Journal of General Practice*, 54, 171–176.

Speck, P., Higginson, I. and Addington-Hall, J. (2004) Spiritual needs in health care, *British Medical Journal*, 329 (7458), 123–124.

Woods, S. (1998) A theory of holism for nursing, *Medicine, Healthcare and Philosophy*, 1, 255–261.

Zaider, T. and Kissane, D. (2007) Resilient families, in Oliviere, D. and Monroe, B. (eds) *Resilience in Palliative Care: Achievement in Adversity*. Oxford: Oxford University Press.

Further reading

Walker, L. (1999) Is integrative science necessary to improve nursing practice? *Western Journal of Nursing Research*, 21 (1), 94–102.

Weiss, S., Haber, J., Horowitz, J., Stuart, G. and Wolfe, B. (2009) The inextricable nature of mental and physical health: implications for integrative care, *Journal of the American Psychiatric Nurses Association*, 15 (6), 371–382.

2

COMMUNICATION IN NURSING
Relating to the Whole Person

Learning outcomes

By the end of this chapter, you should be able to:

- understand the concepts and knowledge underlying communication in nursing;
- analyse the process of communication;
- communicate effectively with patients and their carers, encouraging the open expression of concerns and feelings, and eliciting information for assessment;
- communicate with patients and their carers in a self-reflective manner, responding to changing needs and circumstances, integrating emotional and technical aspects of nursing care.

Introduction

Communication is fundamental to good nursing care. It is a complex integration of social, cultural, behavioural and verbal elements. These include the ability to give information, ask questions and listening actively. High-quality care is based on the ability to communicate effectively, and to integrate communication with the physical and more technical aspects of care. The patient is a significant contributor to the communication process, and problems may arise where the nurse blocks their efforts to communicate their needs and feelings.

What is communication?

Communication is such a basic human activity that it is easy to take it for granted. In reality, it is a very complex activity that is hard to define effectively. At its most basic level, it is a transmission or exchange of information. How we understand this will depend on a number of factors, including the purpose of the communication, the way it is expressed, in terms of both language and behaviour, the extent to which the participants share common language and understandings, and the effects of the context within which communication takes place. Also, we can understand communication

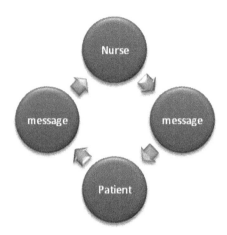

Figure 2.1 Nurse–patient dialogue: a circular process

in terms of specific skills or as groups of skills that together can be understood as communication strategies, for example counselling skills [see Chapter 5] (Chant et al 2002).

As there is always a degree of interaction between people, human communication is best understood as a circular process or as a dialogue (see Figure 2.1).

These messages are expressed in different ways. Of course, this includes words, but non-verbal messages are frequently transmitted by behaviours such as facial expressions and gestures. Messages that are recognized as having a shared meaning within a social context can be termed *cues*, and these may be heard (a pause in speech or a change of tone), seen (e.g. a smile, a gesture of the hand), or felt (a touch); see Chapter 4.

There will also be both internal and external factors that impact on dialogue. Within the context of nurse–patient communication, these will include the following.

Dialogue – internal factors (i.e. within the person)

• Aims, intentions and expectations about the communication; for example, if the nurse feels the priority is to give an important message rather than listen to the patient.

• Understanding of own role within the communication; for example, if the nurse feels they are there to give practical care and not to provide emotional support.

• Knowledge and personal experience of health and illness; for example, the patient may be very familiar with their condition so know what the priorities are in dialogue with the nurse.

• Attitudes towards communication and what it can achieve; for example, if the patient feels they are never listened to so what is the point?

• Skills, confidence and the ability to communicate (nurses who lack confidence may avoid communication whenever possible).

In all of the above, there will be differences between the patient and the nurse. The nurse may be constrained or empowered by their role, whereas the patient may lack confidence in how they can communicate. The patient will have direct personal experience of the illness, but may have less specialist knowledge. The ability to communicate may be affected by their physical and mental condition, including any disability. Both parties may have similar or different goals in communicating, but factors both within the individual and the process of communication may aid or impede effective communication (Feldman-Stewart et al 2005).

Box 2.1 Communication or relationships?

Some nurse theorists have stated that communication between nurses and patients cannot be understood outside of the relationship within which it takes place. This perspective emphasizes the difference between *mechanistic communication*, developed through communication skills, and relationship, developed through the *relational capacity* of the nurse (Hartrick 1997). Central to this position is the belief that the nurse–patient relationship is a values-based expression of human caring, that is greater than the behaviour of communicating itself. In this book, both processes, communication and relationships, are seen as complementary: effective relationships are based on effective communication, and vice versa.

Dialogue – external factors (i.e. within the situation)

- Language, including whether a common language is shared and both parties are proficient in its use (or use of a third-party interpreter).
- Cultural assumptions about communication (including non-verbal cues), mutual roles and the nature of illness.
- Distractions, including being busy and other demands on the nurse.
- Space and privacy.
- Organizational constraints, including expectations of the work environment about relations between nurses and patients.
- The presence and influence of family and friends, which can ease communication and provide additional information, though they can distract from the needs of the patient if the family have unresolved problems.

Communication in context

One of the defining characteristics of communication in nursing is the complexity of the context within which it takes place. This is particularly true of hospitals, where the complex interprofessional environment makes multiple demands on nurses, and unfamiliar procedures and routines, equipment and technical language can be disorienting for patients and their carers. Hospital wards are very busy places, where communication may be constantly interrupted by phone calls, other patients and staff, and the need to fit in treatments and investigations. Nurses manage groups of patients, rather than just individuals. Nurses therefore need to balance the needs of groups with those of individual patients, often with very different needs. Nursing in the community may have fewer of these demands and distractions, but nurses need to carry out their role while respecting the patient's domestic routine and home environment.

Hospitals and other health care facilities are unique cultural environments where some of the usual conventions of social behaviour are suspended or adapted. Nurses and patients share a degree of physical intimacy during caring procedures that is normally experienced only within very immediate family relationships. Patients experience situations of vulnerability, being undressed, asleep, in pain, incapacity and distress in the care of relative strangers. This unusual environment requires common understandings of roles and expectations, based partly on cultural messages (e.g. by the wearing of a uniform) and partly on continual negotiations between individual nurses and patients (e.g. the nurse asking permission before a procedure). In this way, the interpersonal boundaries between nurse and patient are adjusted in response to their health condition (Edwards 1998).

All health care environments are also part of an organization, and the policies, practices and hierarchies that represent it. Within the global context of nursing with limited resources, increasing demands are made on the nurse to quantify, justify and record communication and activity involving patients. This can impact on care in a number of ways. Nurses may be frustrated in their attempts to provide the best quality care by power relationships within the organization that deny them the freedom to do what they believe is best for their patients. As Wilkinson stated: 'It would seem as if nurses have got the skills to facilitate patients but they will not use them unless the environment they work in is conducive to open communication' (1991: 686). They can also be ground down by workload, ongoing demands and lack of support. This can result in demoralization, and even burnout (see Chapter 3). Some of these factors are consistent across different cultural contexts (Park and Song 2005; Anoosheh et al 2009). The effects of the care context in inhibiting communication are summarized below.

Context of care: factors inhibiting communication

- Type of role, and demand on role (e.g. multifunctioning).
- Inadequate staffing levels.
- Heavy workloads and unpredictability of demand.
- Interruptions and distractions, lack of time.
- Environmental constraints (e.g. buildings, space, resources).
- Workplace policies and practices.
- Hierarchies and occupational culture.
- Stress, burnout and lack of support structures.

(Waterworth et al 1999; Chant et al 2002)

Creating a positive environment for effective communication

In spite of these potential constraints, the hospital environment can be adapted to provide a positive context for communication. Privacy, protected space and time can be made available for effective communication. This can facilitate a more 'domestic' or 'homely' environment, where respect is explicitly shown for personal space, promoting comfort and trust (Savage 1995). Similarly, reduction of noise, providing suitable lighting and temperature, and having family carers around are conducive to good communication (Park and Song 2005).

Clarity of roles and expectations helps to prevent confusion, and clear messages should be given about the amount of time available for communicating with patients and their carers. Longer periods of time enable more stable relationships to be built up. In contrast, in the Accident and Emergency Department, most contacts are brief and may therefore be open to greater ambiguity (Baillie 2005). The allocation of specific nurses to patients, and a focus on client-centred care, promotes individualized care, continuity and mutual understanding. Training and support for communication, and policies that support this can all have a positive effect on nurse–patient communication.

Reflection point

This exercise can be done alone but will also work well if you do it with a colleague. Consider your working environment, and make some notes. In your workplace, do any of the following factors hinder effective communication:

- The physical environment?
- Staffing levels or the way that work is organized?
- Policies or any other organizational or managerial factors?
- The nature of your role and the demands made on it?
- The amount of support available to you?

Now consider each of the problem areas that you have identified. What do you think you could do to improve communication within your working environment? How much of this could you achieve yourself and what would you need help with to change?

The patient's contribution to communication

Given that nurse–patient communication is a two-way process, conducted in the interests of the patient, then the patient's perception of the process is very important. Much of the research into nurse–patient communication or nurse–patient interaction (NPI) has neglected the patient's perspective (Jarrett and Payne 1995). Research conducted on what patients value in their interactions with nurses suggests that human qualities such as friendliness, humour, openness and warmth are very important (McCabe 2004). Patients value a genuine interest in them as individuals, and not care based on assumptions about patients in general. Also, indicating availability, displaying competence and providing information, along with good verbal and non-verbal communication skills, are valued aspects of nursing behaviour (Bailey and Wilkinson 1998; Williams and Irurita 2004).

McCabe (2004) makes the important point that the use by nurses of friendliness and humour in social interactions can be done relatively briefly. That is, restricted availability in terms of time does not stop the nurse from engaging with the patient in a meaningful way. Similarly, Bottorff and Morse's research into NPI revealed that 'Nurses were found to interact with patients for relatively brief periods. Nevertheless, they were able to interact on very personal levels' (1994: 59). Patients appear to value both warm interpersonal skills in the nurse, and their ability to carry out the necessary tasks for patient care, even when these take up time that could otherwise be used for social interaction (McCabe 2004). The particular skill of effective nursing is to balance these two major aspects of the work: human caring skills and technical competence. These points are summarized in Box 2.2.

Box 2.2 The qualities of a good nurse communicator that are valued by patients

- Professional, capable and knowledgeable
- Approachable, warm and attentive
- Good verbal and non-verbal skills

It is important to recognize that patients also have a role in managing communication. Although it has been identified that patients have less power within the health care system than the nurse, nonetheless, they are in a position to influence and at times control the process of communication (Hewison 1995; Shattel 2004). They may do this by giving cues to what they do and do not want to talk about. This is one way that they can manage the boundaries of nurse–patient interaction. Patients may have ideas about what they should manage themselves or with their family rather than 'bother' the nurses. They may also be responding to cues from the nurses about being busy or not feeling comfortable dealing with emotional issues, keeping to safe topics that both of them can handle (Jarrett and Payne 1995). There are other factors that can inhibit the patient, preventing their communicating (Box 2.3). These can be overcome with clear, straightforward communication, directly addressing speech and hearing problems, and by effective psychological support and symptom management.

Box 2.3 Factors in the patient that inhibit communication

- Not sharing a common language or lacking confidence, for example, with technical medical language
- Hearing impairment
- Speech or expressive problems
- Anxiety

- Depression
- Pain
- Fatigue
- Weakness
- Malaise
- Poor concentration
- Confusion
- Distress and emotional problems

Non-verbal communication

Non-verbal communication has a significant place in nursing as a practical caring profession. A lot of non-verbal communication is not conscious, so nurses often carry it out without realizing. However, there is evidence that experienced nurses are aware that they communicate non-verbally and use this in a skilled way (Savage 1995; Kozlowska and Doboszynska 2012). Consciously used non-verbal communications in nursing include eye contact, facial expression and touch (Kozlowska and Doboszynska 2012). Non-verbal messages are transmitted by various cues, including gestures, how the body is positioned or presented, and the way in which things are said, *paralanguage* (see Box 2.4). As non-verbal communication includes a range of both conscious and unconscious behaviours, it can be understood as *implicit behaviour*, that is, behaviour within which meaning may be understood without being explicitly stated (Mehrabian 2007).

Box 2.4 Types of non-verbal communication

- Eye contact
- Facial expression (e.g. smiling)
- Head and hand gestures (e.g. nodding)
- Body position, orientation, movements and posture
- Interpersonal space or proximity
- Touch
- Clothing, including uniform, and other aspects of presentation (e.g. perfume)
- Paralanguage (how things are said: speech rate, volume, tone, pitch, pauses, interruptions)

Non-verbal often accompanies verbal communication, and puts it into context; for example, by emphasizing a point with a smile, a frown or hand gestures. The primary effects of non-verbal communication are to convey emotion, and other social effects like turn-taking in conversation. It can represent the emotional content of an interaction even when people are not aware of this or they aim to suppress their emotions.

Because of the nature of signs and cues given in communication, like facial expressions or eye contact, even very brief interactions can communicate a lot of emotional content (Roter et al 2006).

Conveying emotion with non-verbal behaviour

Many verbal interactions in health care focus on the exchange of information, for example, in assessment or giving information, but emotional or affective communication also takes place at the same time. In assessment, eye contact enhances listening skills, so it aids the appraisal of distress. When general practitioners (GPs) give more eye contact, their consultations tend to be longer, involve more talking, and a greater disclosure of psychosocial issues (Bensing et al 1995). Patients report that eye contact makes them feel valued (Williams and Irurita 2004).

Empathy and compassion can be expressed verbally, for example, by encouraging words, or non-verbally by eye contact and facial expression. Bensing et al (1995) suggest that genuine empathy requires congruence between verbal and non-verbal behaviour. For example, a blank expression coupled with words of comfort may not be experienced as comforting by the patient. Interestingly, studies have shown that discordance between comforting words and anxiety in a doctor's voice can actually be perceived as positive by patients. This is probably because it conveys genuine personal concern on the part of the doctor that overrides their professional demeanour (Roter et al 2006). Although non-verbal behaviour is good at conveying comforting emotions, it can also convey more difficult emotions like anger and disapproval. Non-verbal communication skills are not generally taught on nursing or medical courses, but it is possible to develop a raised awareness of them through education (Ishikawa et al 2010). Education that also develops self-awareness is likely to result in a more reflective and sensitive approach to patient care, and more conscious and skilled use of non-verbal communication.

Positioning and posture

Because of the physical activity involved in the process of nursing care, there are opportunities to use the position and posture of the nurse as a means of communication. Savage's (1995) ethnographic study of a specialist nursing unit identified a number of ways that nurses used both touch and the positioning of their bodies in a deliberate and therapeutic way. Often this meant adopting a similar position or eye level to the patient (by sitting or squatting), or presenting a relaxed or open posture. This had the effect of showing interest and availability and promoting conversation, and created a more domestic and less clinical atmosphere.

The use of body position or orientation, posture and interpersonal space, combined with facial expression and eye contact, has the potential to be either threatening or comforting to the patient. It is therefore something to be considered in all nurse–patient interactions. Box 2.5 outlines the potential effects of body position in nursing care.

Box 2.5 Body position in nursing care		
Position	**Example**	**Meaning**
Interpersonal space	0–18 inches	Intimacy, concern *or* threat
	18 inches–4 feet	Personal engagement and interest, availability
	4 feet +	Social engagement, respect for patient's personal space, *or* disengagement
Orientation	Face to face	Concern and personal engagement *or* threat
	At an angle	Availability, respect *or* avoidance
	Above	Authority *or* power
	Same level or below	Respect, empathy
Posture	Closed (e.g. arms crossed)	Tension, defensiveness, anger
	Open	Availability, relaxation, empathy

Cultural differences in non-verbal communication

It is important to recognize that different cultures interpret body gestures, posture and interpersonal space in different ways. The interpersonal space indicated in Box 2.5 represents the norm in many Western cultures but other cultures have closer norms for personal and social space. Also, cultures vary in the extent to which communication favours the implicit or explicit aspects of communication behaviour, with the more explicit and verbal aspects of communication emphasized in Western cultures like the United Kingdom and North America (Burgoon et al 2010). *Gender and power relationships* also impact on communication. For example, eye contact is avoided in some cultures between people of different social status or different genders as a mark of respect (Anoosheh et al 2009).

Reflection point

Have you ever encountered an unexpected or unexplained problem of communication with someone from a different culture? Do any of the factors in Box 2.5 help you understand what might have happened?

Touch

Touch is an essential part of most nursing practice. A distinction is usually made between touch necessary for the achievement of specific nursing tasks, *instrumental touch*, and *expressive touch* that conveys an emotional or caring message (Routasalo 1999). In addition, some nurses believe touch can have intrinsic value as a healing or therapeutic activity, *therapeutic touch* (Meehan 1998). However, while there is evidence that touch promotes feelings of calmness and comfort, there is limited evidence that it has specific healing effects (Routasalo 1999). Most nurses and patients feel comfortable with instrumental touch. It is the most common form of touch in health care, and it is accepted as necessary in hospital and when patients are ill (Edwards 1998). Although different norms are accepted in hospitals, patients and nurses find more personal areas of the body less comfortable to touch or be touched, including the face and sexual organs (Gleeson and Timmins 2005).

Attitudes to expressive touch vary between individuals according to various factors, including personal experience, gender, age and context. Expressive touch may be a spontaneous show of affection; for example, a light touch on the arm to show empathy. In other cases, it may be more deliberate and seen as part of the emotional care of a patient; for example, holding their hand as an explicit act of comfort or caring (Kozlowska and Doboszynska 2012). However well intentioned, touch is not always welcomed, and care should always be exercised when using it in an expressive way, identifying whether it is an acceptable form of communication with the individual patient (Gleeson and Timmins 2005).

Being with a person in distress and sharing an experience with them is another way that nurses can provide comfort and support. *Nursing presence* has been identified as an interpersonal caring activity that has potential benefits for both patient and nurse. Benefits for the patients can be both physical and psychological and include a sense of support, comfort, affirmation and the alleviation of distress (McMahon and Christopher 2011). Presence does not necessarily involve words or touch, but could be simply sitting or staying with the person in distress in silence, if they request it.

Reflection point

Do you regularly use touch as a form of emotional expression in your work? Is this something that you feel comfortable with? How do you know when a patient appreciates this and when they do not?

Verbal communication

Verbal communication is generally better understood and has been more extensively researched than non-verbal communication. Much of the research has identified problems in nurse–patient communication. There are also similar lessons to be learned from the literature on communication between doctors and patients. However, there is a lot of evidence about the most effective forms of verbal communication.

Basic verbal communication skills

The basic skill of verbal communication is engaging in dialogue with the patient (see Box 2.6). This means speaking, listening and responding in a purposeful way. Your own speech needs to be formulated to most effectively express what you mean to say or need to know and your listening needs to be active and attentive. This includes allowing pauses and silences when the patient is thinking or considering their response to you. The extent to which this is achievable within any given situation depends on the amount of time available, the condition of the patient and the context within which it takes place. If communication is ineffective it is likely to cause stress for both the nurse and patient. Effective communication requires confidence. This is often based on experience, but specific communication skills training will also help to develop confidence in communicating and to reduce stress (Wilkinson et al 2008).

Communication is generally more effective if people feel at ease. The use of informal language and everyday social dialogue (e.g. *'how are you today?'*) can help people to feel more relaxed and render the environment less clinical (McCabe 2004). Humour is also an effective way to lighten the mood and reduce the patient's sense of vulnerability (Savage 1995; McCabe 2004). Verbal expressions of empathy or concern also help to create a supportive atmosphere and reinforce the non-verbal expression of empathy through physical caring (Stajduhar et al 2010). This can include statements that legitimize or normalize the patient's feelings or experience, making them feel that their experience is a normal or understandable reaction (Langewitz et al 2010).

Box 2.6 Basic verbal communication skills

- Dialogue (two-way conversation):
  - Giving information, asking questions
  - Active listening and responding
- Informal social conversation
- Humour
- Verbal expressions of empathy

Asking questions and using assessment skills

The skilled use of questions to elicit information is an essential feature of effective communication. Within a conversation, it is helpful to ask an *open question* initially, then use more *focused questions* to clarify the patient's meaning (see Boxes 2.7 and 2.8).

Box 2.7 Using questions to focus a conversation

Nurse: How are you feeling today?

Patient: Oh, not bad, I slept better last night, but I still have some discomfort in my stomach.

Nurse: You had a better night, I am pleased. But you still have some discomfort? Can you tell me what that is like?

Patient: Well, it is a sort of dull pain.

Nurse: So you have a dull pain in your stomach, can you tell me where?

<table>
<tr><td colspan="3" align="center">**Box 2.8 Types of questions**</td></tr>
<tr><td>**Type of question**</td><td>**Example**</td><td>**Use**</td></tr>
<tr><td>Open question</td><td>How are you today?</td><td>To get the patient's perspective</td></tr>
<tr><td>Focused question</td><td>So, does that mean you still have pain?</td><td>Seeking clarification or more information</td></tr>
<tr><td>Closed question</td><td>Are you in pain?</td><td>To get a yes or no answer</td></tr>
<tr><td>Leading question</td><td>You are in pain, aren't you?</td><td>To confirm your own assumption</td></tr>
</table>

Closed questions (eliciting a yes or no answer) have a role in this process, but asking closed questions prematurely prevents the patient from giving information from their perspective, and may simply confirm an existing assumption on the part of the nurse. *Reflection* back to the patient of what they have said summarizes and also enables clarification.

Overall, in terms of patient-focused dialogue, effective verbal behaviours are those that encourage the patient to disclose information about how they feel, and then clarify and obtain detail about this (see Box 2.9). Ineffective verbal behaviours are those that prevent or block disclosure on the part of the patient, or divert the conversation away from significant issues for the patient (see Box 2.10). These ineffective behaviours often serve the function of keeping communication brief (because of time constraints), focused on the nurse's agenda rather than the patient's (because the nurse feels under pressure), or protecting the nurse from emotional issues that they feel uncomfortable or inadequately prepared to deal with.

Box 2.9 Effective verbal communication behaviours

- Open questions
- Focusing
- Probing
- Reflecting
- Paraphrasing
- Clarifying
- Confronting
- Exploring
- Using educated guesses
- Summarizing
- Closing

(Moore et al 2009)

Box 2.10 Ineffective verbal communication behaviours

- Closed questions or leading questions
- Focus on the physical to the exclusion of psychological issues
- Premature or false reassurance
- Advising
- Blaming
- Judging (e.g. *well, you shouldn't have overdone it yesterday...*)
- Changing the topic
- Being defensive
- Rationalizing
- Placating (e.g. *yes of course, it is a nuisance, isn't it?*)
- Interrupting
- Using multiple questions at once (e.g. *how are you today, still in pain?*)

(Moore et al 2009)

Giving information

Information-giving is an essential and commonplace form of communication in nursing. This can include both the giving of significant health-related information to help the patient understand their condition and giving details of procedures so that the patient feels comfortable. In either case, a number of important principles should guide the information-giving process:

- Considering the patient's condition and the timing and format of the information to be given;
- Finding out what the patient already knows;
- Clarifying the reason for giving the information;
- Giving the information in a clear and unambiguous way;
- Allowing time for the patient to consider the information and respond, including asking their own questions;
- Dealing with any questions and gaps in knowledge identified by the patient;
- Identifying how the patient can get more information or ask further questions if they need to (including, for example, paper- or internet-based resources).

Where there is significant news, for example a change or worsening of the patient's condition, or *breaking bad news*, then it is important to consider how this information will be received, and how it will impact on them and their family. In this case, further consideration should be given to:

- ensuring privacy and adequate time for the meeting;
- giving the information in the presence of a family member or friend;

- being clear about the serious nature of the information;
- allowing time and space and encouraging the expression of emotions;
- arranging a follow-up meeting to discuss it if it is felt to be necessary.

Patients appreciate it when professionals allow them time to deal with new information, are able to acknowledge when they are afraid, provide a balance of honesty and hope, and are also able to acknowledge the limits of their own knowledge (Stajduhar et al 2010).

Dealing with emotional issues

A particular characteristic of ineffective communication is blocking statements by changing the subject or moving the conversation away from personal or emotional issues that are important to the patient (Wilkinson 1991). Factors that have been identified that underlie blocking behaviours include: fear of being unable to deal with emotional outbursts from the patient, not wishing to cause distress, uncomfortable personal feelings about death and dying, and feeling under stress. Nurses may be reluctant to 'open a can of worms' if they do not know how to deal with them. Discomfort in dealing with difficult emotional communications can be a feature of staff distancing themselves from patients, and experiencing higher levels of stress and burnout (Gysels et al 2004).

Research into communication skills training in the field of cancer care has shown that participants in several studies developed an enhanced ability to make empathic statements, elicit patients' concerns and discuss their emotions (Gysels et al 2004; Moore et al 2009). Greater capability in these areas is likely to lead to fewer blocking behaviours and more confidence in dealing with strong emotions. However, it remains to be seen whether these changes can be transferred into practice in the longer term. There is some evidence that supervision and support in practice make a difference to this. In dealing with emotional aspects of communication, it is important to bear the following in mind:

- Emotional issues are the most difficult aspect of communication and some nurses actively block emotional communications from patients.
- Greater awareness of our own fears and anxieties as nurses can help to overcome this.
- Nurses need skills in both finding out about patients' emotions and in dealing with them.
- Communication skills training and supervision can help develop skills and confidence.

Reflection point

What do you find the most difficult aspects of communicating with patients and their carers? What has helped you most in dealing with these difficult areas? Have you had access to communication skills training and how has this helped? Make a list of the areas of communication that you would like to develop, and discuss with a colleague, or your manager, how you could develop your skills further.

Telephone and written communication

Increasingly, interactions between nurses and patients are by phone, and email and texting are also becoming a feature of health care. One example of this is *telephone triage*, an assessment of priority for treatment or further assessment, often also giving advice. This system gives rapid access to specialist advice from the patient's home. Other telephone contacts may be initiated by the nurse for assessment of an ongoing health problem in a patient at home. Again, it is likely to involve a two-way exchange of information: gathering data for assessment and giving information or advice. The advantage of telephone contact is its immediacy, but it can present problems as it removes most of the key non-verbal elements of communication, apart from paralanguage, and reduces awareness of context. This necessitates a focus on clear verbal communication, attentive listening, establishing rapport and recording details (by audio-recording or written notes or documentation; see Box 2.11). Patients generally express satisfaction with telephone conversations if they feel their concerns have been recognized and responded to and that enough time has been offered to them (Derkx et al 2009).

Box 2.11 Key elements of telephone communication

- Clarify the names and roles of both parties, including relationship to the patient if they cannot speak on the phone.
- Allow enough time to establish rapport and build a picture of the home context of the patient or caller.
- Listen for paralinguistic elements of communication like tone and pauses.
- Clarify the main concerns that the caller has.
- Speak clearly and concisely when providing information.
- Check regularly for understanding and summarize.
- Ensure there is a clear understanding of the next step for the patient, and how the next contact will be made.
- Document the call including a summary of the main points.

Like telephone conversations, written communication lacks non-verbal elements; it also lacks paralanguage, and provides limited awareness of context. There is a need for clear, unambiguous communication in writing, but care also needs to be taken in achieving the *tone* that the writer wants to convey. For example, a brief, direct message can be interpreted as rude or disrespectful. It is always a good idea to supplement email correspondence with a face-to-face or phone conversation where possible. On the other hand, email also offers the possibility of including links, pictures and other information.

Summary

Effective communication is the key to nursing care. This includes an awareness of the process and context of nursing, and is greatly enhanced by self-awareness. Communication both underlies the provision of physical aspects of care, and is itself a form of nursing care. This nurse–patient interaction has even greater capacity for development where the relationship itself is the focus and this is explored in the next chapter.

Key points

- The social and cultural context has a significant effect on communication in health care.
- Communication is a two-way process and the contribution of the patient is significant.
- Non-verbal communication is very important in nursing and has considerable potential to convey emotional messages, though meanings are often implicit.
- Verbal communication skills have been well defined and effective verbal communication greatly enhances nursing care.
- Verbal and non-verbal communication work together and a reflective, self-aware approach to nursing can make communication more responsive to patients' needs.

References

Anoosheh, M., Zarkhah, S., Faghihzadeh, S. and Vaismoradi, M. (2009) Nurse–patient communication barriers in Iranian nursing, *International Nursing Review*, 56 (2), 243–249.

Bailey, K. and Wilkinson, S. (1998) Communication issues. Patients' views on nurses' communication skills: a pilot study, *International Journal of Palliative Nursing*, 4 (6), 300–305.

Baillie, L. (2005) An exploration of nurse–patient relationships in accident and emergency, *Accident and Emergency Nursing*, 13, 9–14.

Bensing, J., Kerssens, J. and van der Pasch, M. (1995) Patient-directed gaze as a tool for discovering and handling psychosocial problems in general practice, *Journal of Nonverbal Behavior*, 19 (4), 223–242.

Bottorff, J. and Morse, J. (1994) Identifying types of attending: patterns of nurses' work, *IMAGE: Journal of Nursing Scholarship*, 26 (1), 53–60.

Burgoon, J., Guerrero, L. and Floyd, K. (2010) *Nonverbal Communication*. London: Allyn & Bacon.

Chant, S., Jenkinson, T., Randle, J. and Russell, G., (2002) Communication skills: some problems in nursing education and practice, *Journal of Clinical Nursing*, 11, 12–21.

Derkx, H., Rethans, J-J., Maiburg, B., Winkens, R., Muijtjens, A., van Rooij, H. and Knottnerus, A. (2009) Quality of communication during telephone triage at Dutch out-of-hours centre, *Patient Education and Counselling*, 74, 174–178.

Edwards, S. (1998) An anthropological interpretation of nurses' and patients' perceptions of the use of space and touch, *Journal of Advanced Nursing*, 28 (4), 809–817.

Feldman-Stewart, D., Brundage, M. and Tishelman, C. (2005) A conceptual framework for patient–professional communication: an application to the cancer context, *Psycho-oncology*, 14, 801–809.

Gleeson, M. and Timmins, F. (2005) A review of the use and clinical effectiveness of touch as a nursing intervention, *Clinical Effectiveness in Nursing*, 9, 69–77.

Gysels, M., Richardson, A. and Higginson, I. (2004) Communication training for health professionals who care for patients with cancer: a systematic review of effectiveness, *Journal of Supportive Care in Cancer*, 12 (10), 692–700.

Hartrick, G. (1997) Relational capacity: the foundation for interpersonal nursing practice, *Journal of Advanced Nursing*, 26, 523–528.

Hewison, A. (1995) Nurses' power in interactions with patients, *Journal of Advanced Nursing*, 21, 75–82.

Ishikawa, H., Hashimoto, H. and Kinoshita, E. (2010) Can nonverbal communication skills be taught? *Medical Teacher*, 32, 860–863.

Jarrett, N. and Payne, S. (1995) A selective review of the literature on nurse–patient communication: has the patient's contribution been neglected? *Journal of Advanced Nursing*, 22, 72–78.

Kozlowska, L. and Doboszynska, A. (2012) Nurses' nonverbal methods of communicating with patients in the terminal phase, *International Journal of Palliative Nursing*, 18 (1), 40–46.

Langewitz, W., Heydrich, L., Nübling, M., Szirt, L., Weber, H. and Grossman, P. (2010) Swiss Cancer League communication skills training programme for oncology nurses: an evaluation, *Journal of Advanced Nursing*, 66 (10), 2266–2277.

McCabe, C. (2004) Nurse–patient communication: an exploration of patients' experiences, *Journal of Clinical Nursing*, 13, 41–49.

McMahon, M. and Christopher, K. (2011) Towards a mid-range theory of nursing presence, *Nursing Forum*, 46 (2), 71–82.

Meehan, T. (1988) Therapeutic touch as a nursing intervention, *Journal of Advanced Nursing*, 28 (1), 117–125.

Mehrabian, A. (2007) *Nonverbal Communication*. London: Aldine Transaction.

Moore, P., Wilkinson, S. and Mercado, R. (2009) Communication skills training for health care professionals working with cancer patients, their families and/or carers (review), *The Cochrane Library*, 2009, Issue 1.

Park, E. and Song, M. (2005) Communication barriers perceived by older patients and nurses, *International Journal of Nursing Studies*, 42, 159–166.

Roter, D., Frankel, R., Hall, J. and Sluyter, D. (2006) The expression of emotion through nonverbal behaviour in medical visits, *Journal of General Internal Medicine*, 21, S28–S34.

Routasalo, P. (1999) Physical touch in nursing studies: a literature review, *Journal of Advanced Nursing*, 30 (4), 843–850.

Savage, J. (1995) *Nursing Intimacy*. London: Scutari Press.

Shattel, M. (2004) Nurse-patient interaction: a review of the literature, *Journal of Clinical Nursing*, 13, 714–722.

Stajduhar, K., Thorne, S., McGuinness, L. and Kim-Sung, C. (2010) Patient perceptions of helpful communication in the context of advanced cancer, *Journal of Clinical Nursing*, 19, 2039–2047.

Waterworth, S., May, C. and Luker, K. (1999) Clinical 'effectiveness' and 'interrupted' work, *Clinical Effectiveness in Nursing*, 3, 163–169.

Wilkinson, S. (1991) Factors which influence how nurses communicate with cancer patients, *Journal of Advanced Nursing*, 16, 677–688.

Wilkinson, S., Perry, R. and Blanchard, K. (2008) Effectiveness of a three-day communication skill course in changing nurses' communication skills with cancer/palliative care patients: a randomised controlled trial, *Palliative Medicine*, 22, 365–375.

Williams, A. and Irurita, V. (2004) Therapeutic and non-therapeutic interpersonal interactions: the patient's perspective, *Journal of Clinical Nursing*, 13, 806–815.

3

PSYCHOSOCIAL NURSING CARE
Caring for the Whole Person

Learning outcomes

By the end of this chapter, you should be able to:

- understand the nature of caring and nurse–patient interaction;
- develop an awareness of the nature of closeness and involvement in the nurse–patient relationship;
- analyse theory underlying the practice of therapeutic relationships in nursing;
- develop a capacity for self-awareness, self-reflection and self-management.

Introduction

Nursing interactions with patients have unique qualities, and there are considerable opportunities for further developing nursing's therapeutic role. This can be achieved by engaging with patients in ways that are meaningful for them, and that acknowledge issues of closeness and intimacy in the nurse–patient relationship. However, this work also makes emotional demands on the nurse, and the nurse needs to develop self-awareness and strategies for self-management.

Psychosocial nursing care

Nurses spend long periods of time being with or being available to patients, and providing care. However, despite this being such a common activity, the nature of nursing care remains controversial and there is not universal agreement about what it is (or what it is not!). Much of the debate is about the nature of caring, and what this involves. The terms *being with* and *doing for* are often used as shorthand for the acts of comforting presence and providing physical care that are characteristic of nursing.

Some studies have compared nurses' views on what caring behaviours are with the views of patients, and these usually show differences of perception. Nurses tend to rate expressive or interpersonal behaviours (like listening) more highly than patients, who value skilled, knowledgeable nurses, and there is some evidence that this is consistent across different cultures (Papstavrou et al 2011).

There are a number of reasons why this difference in perception may occur. Patients may value their immediate recovery from illness over other, interpersonal, aspects of care. Nurses, in turn, may take their basic competence for granted, and focus on what they consider the more therapeutic or satisfying aspects of their role. It is also likely that the implicit value of some caring behaviours is not recognized by patients: nursing can be seen as a *moral* rather than a *technical* activity. However, it is clear that patients do value the interpersonal aspects of nursing, if they are carried out by nurses who also demonstrate knowledge and skill in the practical aspects of nursing.

This area of research highlights an important point: nurses need to be clear what their patients' needs and priorities are, in addition to their own professional values and priorities. Caring, then, must involve a significant engagement with the patient's perception of their own needs. This can only be achieved through the interpersonal aspects of nursing care, but this needs to move beyond communication skills alone. Consider the following conversation between a nurse and patient.

Example: nurse–patient interaction

Patient: I had a terrible time when I was recovering from surgery. I was in so much pain, and I couldn't even go to the toilet without help. I felt like I had lost all of my independence.

Nurse: The most important thing now is that we get your symptoms under control and we can help you to make a full recovery.

Patient: I don't like feeling dependent on people. It's even worse than the pain. But together they made me feel so vulnerable, like I had no control over anything in my life any more.

Nurse: Is your pain controlled now?

Patient: Yes, I am taking painkillers and they are controlling the pain, thank you.

Nurse: Good, we can give you stronger analgesia if necessary.

In the scenario above, the nurse is listening and responding effectively, doing her job of supporting the patient to recover from surgery. However, there are messages that the patient is giving about the meaning attached to her experience of surgery, which the nurse either is missing or does not feel it is important to respond to. The nurse is certainly not doing anything wrong, but she is missing an opportunity to understand the patient's perspective better. We return to this conversation later in this chapter, seeing how it could be managed in a way that encourages the patient to share their feelings and personal meanings about their experience.

The manner in which the patient is invited to share their perspective is significant. Where possible, this should move beyond a simple sharing of information to an invitation to share a *narrative*; that is, a more detailed account of how the patient is feeling in their own terms, involving their significant others, and with an expression of the emotion and meaning attached to events. Psychosocial nursing care can then be based on an integration of the patient's personal perspective and the nurse's professional perspective.

Reflection point

What do you feel are the most important features of the nursing care that you provide? Consider how much the following have influenced your approach to nursing care: your training and continuing education, your personal values, the influence of nursing peers and people you respect, feedback from patients.

Nurse–patient interaction

The interaction between nurses and patients has been the subject of much discussion and research. This body of literature is important in understanding the theoretical background to nurse–patient interaction. Hildegard Peplau's book *Interpersonal Relations in Nursing* ([1952] 1988) identified the potential for nursing to be educational and constructive, to aid personal development and living effectively within a community. Peplau and subsequent *interactionist nursing theorists* including King, Orlando, Travelbee and Wiedenbach, emphasized the centrality of nurse–patient interaction to the process of nursing care, drawing on psychodynamic theories and Rogers' client-centred psychology (Kitson 1993).

In order to provide effective care, nurses need to have a certain level of interpersonal competence, developed through social interaction with the patient (Kasch 1986). Fosbinder (1994) identified four key interpersonal processes underlying nurse–patient interaction. These are *translating* (e.g. informing, explaining), *getting to know you* (e.g. being friendly, using humour), *establishing trust* (e.g. being in charge, anticipating needs) and *going the extra mile* (e.g. being a friend, doing the extra). Fosbinder suggested that nurse–patient interaction is a combination of professional confidence and less formal relationship-building skills.

However, some research has suggested that nurse–patient interactions do not meet the needs of patients. For example, studies from the 1980s conducted in oncology (Bond 1983), surgery (Macleod Clark 1983), and in medical and surgical wards (Webster 1981) showed that communication with patients was often superficial, routinized and task-related, and nurses blocked communications by patients relating to emotional aspects of care. Research conducted during the subsequent decade suggested that these influential studies had been superseded by changes in the quality of nursing, particularly from task-related to patient-centred care (Jarrett and Payne 1995).

Bottorff and Morse (1994) also identified methodological problems with the earlier research. First, they argue that a concentration on verbal interactions devalued non-verbal interaction, particularly touch. Second, they suggest that much of the earlier research had not studied the unique intimacy and complexity of nursing in context. Their research involved the analysis of videotapes of nurses' bedside work, which revealed ways in which nurses made themselves available to patients, or *types of attending*. Subsequent research (Bottorff and Varcoe 1995) suggested additional complexity in the form of transitions between types of attending. Nurses shifted between a focus on task and a focus on relationship. This is significant as it involves the skilled use of opportunities to integrate physical and psychosocial care. Earlier criticisms of nurses as lacking communication skills and focusing on physical tasks may have missed the importance of the manner in which these tasks are carried out. What makes nursing unique is its combination of close interpersonal working relationships with physical closeness.

Therapeutic relationships in nursing

This sense of the uniqueness of nursing has led a body of literature on *nursing as therapy*, emphasizing the nurse–patient relationship and also looking for opportunities to develop nursing in both conventional and novel directions (McMahon 1991). The nurse–patient relationship was conceptualized as one involving partnership, intimacy and reciprocity. It also involved education, providing comfort and manipulating the environment for the benefit of the patient. The ethnographic study by Savage (1995) has given us some of the best insights into how this vision of nursing works in practice. She describes nursing relationships involving a unique degree of *closeness* or *intimacy*. This involved the use of touch, humour and metaphor, and the skilful use of interpersonal space. The ward environment was manipulated in ways that rendered it more familiar and 'domestic', and therefore more comfortable and less alienating for the patient.

The patient's perspective on what is therapeutic in the nurse–patient relationship was explored in Williams and Irurita's (2004) grounded theory study of patient's experiences of care. Their main finding was that emotional comfort was the significant factor identified by patients as helping or hindering their recovery. Therapeutic interactions were those that facilitated emotional comfort by enhancing the patients' feelings of personal control, generating feelings of security, knowledge and personal value. Feelings of security were developed by nurses (and other staff) who indicated that they were available and competent, and by taking time to get to know the patients. Providing information helped the patients to feel informed, and their sense of personal value was enhanced by effective non-verbal and verbal communication. Williams and Irurita (2004) suggest that their study demonstrates the interconnectedness of psychosocial and physical aspects of care.

Box 3.1 Summary – nursing as a therapeutic activity

- Promoting a sense of trust and security by demonstrating competence
- Effective non-verbal and verbal communication
- Education and providing information
- The use of metaphor and humour by nurses
- A sense of closeness and intimacy, and partnership with the patient
- Manipulating the environment for the comfort of the patient

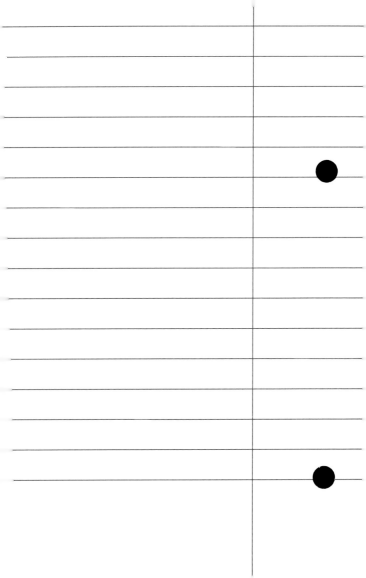

Significant features of therapeutic nursing activity emerge from these accounts (see Box 3.1). Some of these will be explored in more detail in the following sections. The term therapeutic in nursing has also been used to describe the use of specific therapies, including complementary therapies, by nurses. These have included, for example, massage and therapeutic touch. Within this book, complementary therapies are not explored in detail, though there is a discussion of the use of touch in Chapter 2. There is an extended discussion of the potential for developing the *psychotherapeutic* potential of nurses in Chapter 5.

Reflection point

Do you think the nursing care that you provide includes any features that you would describe as *therapeutic nursing* or *nursing as therapy*?

Closeness and involvement

Closeness is frequently cited as characteristic of therapeutic nurse–patient relationships. Peplau (1969) described professional closeness as sharing some elements with social relationships but being distinctive in that it is focused solely on the needs of the patient, and not those of the nurse. In an interview-based study by Ramos (1992), experienced nurses described how they saw their relationships with patients as 'modified social relationships', modified in the sense of being more purposeful and skilled. Closeness in the study by Savage (1995) was described as a form of rapport or understanding, similar to the concept of empathy. This was seen as different from the closeness experienced outside of the hospital in social and family relationships.

The distinct nature of closeness in nursing relationships has also been described in terms of *involvement*. This suggests that relationships built around times of suffering inevitably bring a personal dimension. May's (1991) qualitative study of staff nurses' attitudes towards care of terminally ill patients produced three models of involvement, which represented differing degrees of personal and organizational emphasis. Involvement could be unsatisfactory to both nurses and patients if it was either too personal or not personal enough (see Box 3.2). Relationships can be superficial, or *overinvolved* (Ramos 1992). Another interview-based study of nurses, by Morse (1991), suggests that relationships need to achieve a balance between task and person that can be termed *therapeutic*.

Box 3.2 Models of involvement

- *Primary* involvement represents a balance between personal and organizational objectives, and is generally satisfactory to both nurse and patient
- *Demonstrative* involvement overemphasizes the personal to the extent that excessive emotional demands are made on both nurse and patient
- *Associational* involvement, where organizational demands are met, but patients may not feel adequately involved as people in the process

(May 1991)

In spite of the evidence for nurse–patient involvement, there are several studies that have suggested nurses avoid emotional interactions or distance themselves emotionally from the patient. Menzies Lyth's (1959) influential observational study of nursing concluded that the pain and suffering encountered in clinical situations mirrored internal psychological conflicts in the nurse. This was based on a psychodynamic understanding of nurse–patient interaction. As a result the nurse was at risk of being overwhelmed by anxiety. The response of nursing was the creation of 'social systems', including ritual or routinized tasks and hierarchies, which acted as defences against anxiety, largely by emotional detachment from the individual patient.

Subsequent studies have shown that nurses may avoid and distance themselves from patients (Gysels et al 2004). Roberts and Snowball (1999) identified that closeness, overinvolvement and distancing may be seen as a continuum within the nurse–patient relationship (Box 3.3). Nurses may get more close to patients because they identify with them (e.g. because they are the same age), or lose their professional objectivity and become overinvolved. Alternatively, they may lack the time, confidence or support necessary to engage with patients, and become detached or even distance themselves from emotional contact with patients. The optimum state is one of closeness, based on a professional understanding of the patient's condition. This can be achieved through a balance of the interpersonal and professional aspects of the nurse's role.

Box 3.3 Nurse–patient interpersonal involvement: a continuum	
Level of involvement	**Description**
Overinvolvement	Feeling emotionally involved in a way that makes significant demands on the nurse's emotions. Involvement with a patient to the extent that the nurse treats their needs as more important than, or to the exclusion of, other patients
Identification	Identifying with a patient because of their particular characteristics (e.g. age, family circumstances). This can lead to the nurse feeling, for example, *they are like me*, or *they are like my mother*, and consequently feeling close to them and paying particular attention to them
Closeness	Emotional engagement with a patient that is based on an understanding of their particular needs, and makes nursing care more person-centred and meaningful for both the patient and the nurse
Detachment	Standing back emotionally from the patient, while remaining effective in providing nursing care. The nurse may miss opportunities for developing a deeper, more personal relationship with the patient
Distance	The nurse positively distances herself from the patient(s) and may fail to identify and meet their needs. This may include avoiding contact with them.

Reflection point

Do you have personal experience of feeling more involved with a patient than you were comfortable with? Do you feel that you have ever avoided contact with a patient because of how you felt? Is there anything in particular that you have learned from this experience?

Intimacy and empathy

Intimacy, like closeness, has been described as a feature of therapeutic nursing. It is, however, a more specific and problematic concept. Savage (1995) identifies the unique physical intimacy nurses have with patients, which is often combined with emotional closeness, and points out that this level of intimacy does not normally occur outside of sexual or close family relationships. In a review of the concept of intimacy in nursing, Williams (2001) distinguishes between physical and emotional intimacy. Physical intimacy is an inevitable feature of nursing care when patients are dependent and vulnerable, and it can provide opportunities for emotional closeness if both the nurse and patient are receptive to this.

Psychological or emotional intimacy, on the other hand, has an essential quality of *reciprocity* or sharing of feeling, and this involves *disclosure* on the part of both the nurse and the patient (Williams 2001). Disclosure can make the relationship very personal, so could contribute to overinvolvement. The concept of *empathy* may be a preferable way of understanding the emotional closeness that occurs between the nurse and patient. Empathy can be understood as a capacity to understand another person's current feelings, in a non-judgemental way, and to communicate this understanding to that person (Wiseman 1996). *Sympathy* is different in that it is responding by feeling sorry for the other person, or imagining how we would feel under the same circumstances. Empathy is an important concept in communication (see Chapter 2), and in counselling and psychotherapy (see Chapter 5).

Though it is important, empathy may not be a sufficient basis for understanding the unique potential of the nurse–patient relationship. Kirk (2007) describes a *model of clinical intimacy*, and points out that if intimacy is seen as an interpersonal process, then intimate nurse–patient interactions can take place when the following occur:

1. The patient discloses personally significant information.
2. The nurse is perceived to have responded in a manner that is caring, concerned and validating (a complementary response).
3. Both nurse and patient experience a sense of intimacy as a result.

Importantly, the nurse does not have to disclose their own feelings to achieve this, but their response must be *complementary* to the patient's self-disclosure, rather than *reciprocal*. The following example is the same interaction as we saw earlier in this chapter, but this time the nurse uses disclosure as a way of relating to the patient.

Example: reciprocal response (involving disclosure by the nurse)

Patient: I had a terrible time when I was recovering from surgery. I was in so much pain, and I couldn't even go to the toilet without help. I felt like I had lost all of my independence.

Nurse: Oh how awful. That must have been terrible. I had surgery once and the pain was excruciating. I thought it would never go away.

Patient: Really? How long did your pain last?

Nurse: Well, I had to take painkillers for a month.

Patient: So you must know what I went through?

Nurse: Oh yes, being in pain is just so awful, I can imagine how you felt.

In this interaction, the nurse discloses their own feelings, and this could be complementary, if they use this in a way that demonstrates caring and understanding. On the other hand, if the focus of the interaction switches to their own experience, it will detract from the patient's problems. So, it depends on what would happen next. In the following example, the nurse shows a complementary response.

Example: complementary response

Patient: I had a terrible time when I was recovering from surgery. I was in so much pain, and I couldn't even go to the toilet without help. I felt like I had lost all of my independence.

Nurse: Oh how awful. That must have been terrible. So you were in pain and you felt you had lost your independence?

Patient: Yes, I think it was worse feeling dependent on people. It's even worse than the pain. But together they made me feel so vulnerable, like I had no control over anything in my life any more.

Nurse: Gosh, feeling like you've lost control over your life, that must be difficult. You seem to me such an independent person.

Patient: Yes, that's it, that's me. I am independent and I didn't feel like me any more.

Nurse: Well, you know that I aim to support you in maintaining your independence. You know how to contact me. I would like to know if there is anything that I could do to help you to keep going when you are at home.

In this interaction, the nurse displays both empathy and intimate interaction. Empathy is a capacity for understanding the patient's feelings and the meaning that they make of events. So, understanding what it is like to be a person who values independence but feels they are losing it is an expression of empathy. Intimacy on the other hand allows the nurse to get involved in the process of making meaning with the patient through their complementary responses. This is a significant role for the nurse in the life of the patient, as they encounter diagnoses, symptoms, treatments and changes in their health status. In the exchange above, the response of the nurse enables the patient to reflect on how the illness and treatment have affected their sense of who they are. The nurse's understanding of the effects of illness gives them insights that they can share with the patient; and clarifying their own role in relation to the patient gives them a sense of their needs being understood.

Significantly for contemporary nursing, with all of its pressures and time constraints, *intimate interactions* do not require extensive periods of contact; rather, a willingness and capacity on the part of both patient and nurse to engage in the process. This could involve, for example, holding a patient's hand during a distressing procedure. However, *intimate relationships* between patient and nurse can take place over a longer period of time, where *shared meanings* can be developed in response to events. This could be the case, for example, where a specialist nurse provides continuity of care to a patient or family over a number of weeks, months or even years. In this case, an interaction will be based on existing shared meanings between the patient and nurse.

Example: shared meanings within an interaction

Patient: After I got out of hospital this last time, you know, I was very weak and I needed my husband to help me to go to the toilet. It brought back all of those feelings of vulnerability again, from after my last operation. I felt so frightened. I mean, I even thought, will I ever get better?

Nurse: Yes, I remember that time after your operation. You felt you'd lost your independence, and that wasn't like you. But you did feel you got your independence back.

Patient: Yes, it is so important to me to feel I am not dependent on people. Even my husband. I mean, I want to look after him, not him look after me.

Nurse: But it sounds like you are worried about the future now.

Patient: Yes, I am. I think maybe I'm being a bit silly, but I really worry now that things will never be back to normal.

Nurse: What do you mean by normal?

Patient: Normal. Me being able to do everything I used to. Me being able to look after him without worrying if I will get too tired to do the cleaning.

Nurse: Yes, I can see that your fatigue is a real problem when you want to get on and do your housework, to be your old self again. I would like to help you with some suggestions about how you can manage your tiredness. But it might mean you can't do everything you want to do all of the time.

Patient: Can't I do all the things I used to do?

Nurse: I think you have to get the right balance for you. Plan your time and plan what you do. If you do too much, you will make yourself too tired and then you can't do the things you want to.

In this interaction, the nurse is helping the patient to adjust to changes in their condition, reappraising what can be done in response to feelings of tiredness. Note that the nurse is neither disclosing their own feelings, nor suggesting what is right for the patient. Rather, they are supporting the patient in finding the right level of activity for their current condition, but contributing their own professional perspective on this as well. In this way, the nurse and patient are exploring the meaning of 'independence' and 'normal' for the patient, and how this might be changing.

Meaning and narrative

In working with the meanings that people have about their illness, nurses have a number of potential opportunities and strategies to help the patient. In the interactions above, the nurse was using empathic statements and complementary responses to show understanding and to share meanings with the patient. However, patients do not always develop meaning with the help of a professional. Most of the time they will do this on their own, or with their partner, or with a friend or family member. This will be based on their existing understandings of health and illness, their view of themselves and the world, and in relation to previous life experience.

Narrative is a useful way of thinking about how people understand and communicate their experience of health and illness. Narratives are synonymous with stories though there are some differences (see Chapter 4). A personal narrative will often say something about the patient's perspective on who they are and how they see themselves, what has happened to them up to now, what their current concerns are and where they see themselves going. *Narrative research* explores personal stories of illness, and this has given us many insights into the nature of the illness experience. This includes the ways in which people construct meaning in the face of suffering, disruption and changing understandings of illness and health. It is the means by which patients seek to understand and normalize their experience. These research narratives, or parts of them, can be categorized according to their prominent themes and underlying plots (see Boxes 3.4 and 3.5).

Box 3.4 Types of illness narrative – Bury (2001)

Contingent narrative   This describes how the illness has affected the person's life in practical ways, how its onset links to other life events, and an exploration of the causation of illness, using medical and lay explanations. The account of the onset of psychosis on page 135 of Chapter 8 is an example.

Moral narrative   This concerns the self-image, sense of moral value and social identity that the person holds, as they change and adapt in response to the illness. For example, could becoming ill be attributed to any fault on their part (like an unhealthy lifestyle), and would loss of independence reflect badly on them as a moral person?

Core narrative   Core narratives explore personal experience in terms of shared cultural meanings around illness and suffering; for example, the tragedy of illness or heroism in the face of illness.

Box 3.5 Types of illness narrative – Frank (1995)

Restitution narrative   This follows a pattern of a normal past, a decline due to ill health in the present, with the hope of recovery in the future. In a study of breast cancer survivors, one tells her story of diagnosis and treatment, and ends with *'I'm just thankful that we have the diagnostic equipment, that it was caught early and I had skilled surgeons, that I'm well'* (Thomas-MacLean 2004: 1650).

Chaos narrative   A chaos narrative envisages life as never improving after illness; the story lacks plot. A participant in the same study as above says '*...I had a biopsy yesterday and that's my third biopsy. Luckily, two of them are fine. This one is 99% okay. I won't know until next week...You know I think this has worried me a bit because I got so I could relax and not think about it and all of a sudden this came up. I thought I could go the whole summer without having to have an appointment for a change with a doctor and this came up'* (Thomas-MacLean 2004: 1653).

Quest narrative   This narrative reframes the disruption of life as a challenge that gives a sense of purpose, with the potential for transformation through the illness journey. As another breast cancer survivor says: '*And, as a result, I've done some things I never would have. I took my first hot air balloon ride last Sunday. It was just simply beautiful...And I've learned to swim'* (Thomas-MacLean 2004: 1654).

Reflection point

Do you think that the *Example: shared meanings within an interaction* on page 47 has any elements of these different types of illness narrative?

Narrative therapy

Another use of narrative is *narrative therapy*. Narratives as a form of therapy have been used in mental health nursing (Gaydos 2005) and end of life care (Noble and Jones 2005). This involves the therapist or nurse listening and supporting the patient in the construction of their narrative, or it can involve groups of patients writing about their experiences (Brown et al 2010). It can be understood as a form of personal storytelling that helps the patient make sense of their experience and construct an autobiographical account of their illness. Illness, particularly chronic illness, can be viewed as *biographical disruption*, or the disturbance of personal identity that is experienced by having a coherent life story. Stories hold the potential for *narrative reconstruction*, that is, repairing the disruption by making sense of what has happened and rebuilding the personal biography (Williams 1984).

It is not always possible to obtain a full narrative account of a patient's experience of illness, even of a symptom. But it is important to know in what form the patient understands their experience, and that this is essentially different from the medical model of illness that is prevalent in health care. Our perspective as nurses, no matter how patient-centred, will never be the same as that of the patient we care for. But we can meet them in a place that affords us insights into their world of meaning, and enables us to jointly construct meanings, when common interest, time and resources allow. As part of the process of assessment, this may enable us to get a glimpse of the patient's world beyond our immediate need for clinical information (see Chapter 4). Box 3.6 summarizes this section of the chapter, comparing the uses of empathy, intimacy and narrative in the nurse–patient relationship.

Box 3.6 Summary: uses of empathy, intimacy, narrative		
	For the patient	**For the nurse**
Empathy	Enables the patient to feel understood and can provide the basis for meeting their needs for care or other forms of therapy	Enables the nurse to gain an understanding of how the patient feels and the nurse can use this as the basis for professional assessment and care or therapy
Intimacy	Helps the patient to develop shared understandings and meanings of events with the nurse	Develops joint understandings and shared meanings with the patient as the basis for an ongoing emotionally engaged professional relationship
Narrative	Develops a personal account of what has happened to them, what it means and how they feel about it. It can be therapeutic for the patient to construct their narrative through dialogue with a nurse, or by writing their account down as a record of their experiences	Provides a detailed account of what has happened to the patient in their own words, what it means to them and how they feel about it. This can be used as a form of assessment and it is also therapeutic for the patient to have their story heard by the nurse

Engagement and emotional work

Humour has frequently been reported in the nursing literature as a feature of nurse–patient relationships. It can be initiated by either the patient or the nurse, and it often has the effect of 'breaking the ice', reducing tensions and ambiguities in the social environment. This can include managing embarrassment over situations of physical intimacy like using a bedpan (Fosbinder 1994). Use of humour is one of the ways that both patients and nurses cope in the face of stress. It can lighten the mood (Savage 1995) and produce a positive emotional state in those who share a joke (McCreaddie and Wiggins 2007). It has a particular role in developing *rapport* between nurses and patients (Savage 1995). This is part of the process of *engagement* that is necessary for the development of the nurse–patient relationship.

Being engaged emotionally makes demands on the nurse as a person. These demands can include emotional involvement, overinvolvement and burnout (or compassion fatigue); role strain, role demand and role ambiguity; balancing emotional and physical intimacy; working with people we either like or dislike; and high moral values and expectations of ourself (see Box 3.7). Other stresses that impact on the nurse include communication within the interprofessional team, problems with management and resources, and a lack of training or support.

Box 3.7 Emotional demands on the nurse	
Emotional demand	**Effects on the nurse**
Emotional involvement	Distress
	Finding it hard to deal with strong feelings at work
	Work affecting home life
Overinvolvement and burnout (or compassion fatigue)	Feeling overwhelmed emotionally
	Feeling unable to disengage from work
	Exhaustion, demoralization
	Loss of interest and motivation
	Self-medication (alcohol, drugs)
	Depression
Role demand, role strain and role ambiguity	Finding the role too demanding
	Conflict with colleagues
	Being uncertain where the role ends
Balancing emotional and physical intimacy	Feeling close to people and also carrying out intimate tasks
	Working with personal feelings of disgust at damaged bodies, body fluids, etc.
Working with people we either like or dislike	Feeling closer to some patients because of their age or other characteristics
	Finding it hard to be professional with people we dislike or who annoy us
High moral values and expectations of self	Difficulty meeting personal expectations
	Disappointment, frustration with self and others

The emotional aspects of the nursing role have been described as *emotional labour*. Emotional labour is an ambiguous term that describes how nurses invest some of themselves as a person, but in a manner that is similar to acting. This can involve either inducing or suppressing feelings to produce a sense of being cared for in the patient

(Smith 1992). So, on the one hand, it makes emotional demands on the person, on the other hand, it has been criticized as nursing without *authenticity*. However, the important point is that the nurse is sincere in their expression of feeling and the patient feels cared for (de Raeve 2002), and there is some overlap between this and the idea of intimacy in nursing.

Self-awareness and self-management in nursing

Being engaged with the patient and managing emotions is central to psychosocial nursing care. This *emotional work* does make demands on the nurse and is not possible without self-management, that is, a capacity to manage both the nurse's own feelings and the emotions that they present to the patient. This in turn requires the development of a capacity for *self-awareness* and *self-reflection* in the nurse. There are a number of strategies that nurses can use to develop this. In this book, *reflection points* pose questions that invite the reader to reflect on their own experiences of providing care. These questions provide a trigger for learning from personal experience.

Reflection can also be done through writing personal reflective accounts or keeping a diary of professional practice. Writing accounts in this way has similarities to constructing a personal narrative. Reflection can also be done with another person, someone who understands your work and its context. This can be through a process of supervision, if that process is focused on developing self-awareness rather than as a managerial process (Severinsson 2001). Just as we should develop resilience in our patients, we need to develop strategies for strengthening our own resilience as nurses and as people (see Box 3.8).

Box 3.8 Strategies for strengthening personal professional resilience

- Building positive nurturing relationships
- Seeing positive benefits in adversity
- Developing emotional insight
- Achieving life balance and spirituality
- Becoming more reflective

(Jackson et al 2007)

Reflection point

Looking at the points in Box 3.8, do you recognize any strategies that you currently use? How do you think you could build personal resilience in yourself as a professional?

Using these strategies and achieving these outcomes is a significant challenge to nurses. Most people enter nursing to serve others, so the idea of self-care can initially seem alien. However, effective nursing can only be carried out by a nurse who has the resilience to survive emotional demands over the period of their career. In addition to developing self-awareness and self-reflection, nurses can enhance their resilience by deliberately seeking to build nurturing relationships in both their personal and their professional life. Professionally, this can include seeking the support and guidance of a mentor, someone with personal qualities, experience and skills that earn the respect of colleagues. The process of supervision can be supportive and educative and provide opportunities for reflection either one to one with the supervisor or in a group setting. Given the very personal nature of nursing, supervision helps to keep a professional focus. Health care organizations also have a responsibility to nurture their staff through positive employment policies, promoting work–life balance and providing support for continuing professional education.

Summary

This chapter has explored the potential for nurses to gain deeper and more meaningful relationships with their patients. It has raised some areas of complexity and challenge, not least the personal emotional demands these relationships make on the nurse. Chapters 2 and 3 have focused on the working relationships of nurse and patient. The next chapter addresses one of the most central elements of nursing care – assessment – and how this can be used to develop care.

Key points

Psychosocial nursing care is nursing that integrates:

- nurse–patient interaction and the therapeutic relationship;
- finding opportunities to optimize the nursing role through closeness and intimacy;
- developing meaning in the patient's and the nurse's experience;
- developing self-awareness and professional growth.

References

Bond, S. (1983) Nurses' communication with cancer patients, in Wilson-Barnett, J. (ed.) *Nursing Research: Ten Studies in Patient Care*. Chichester: John Wiley & Sons, pp. 58–79.

Bottorff, J. and Morse, J. (1994) Identifying types of attending: patterns of nurses' work, *IMAGE: Journal of Nursing Scholarship*, 26 (1), 53–60.

Bottorff, J. and Varcoe, C. (1995) Transitions in nurse–patient interactions: a qualitative ethology, *Qualitative Health Research*, 5 (3), 315–331.

Brown, C., Dick, B. and Berry, R. (2010) How do you write about pain? A preliminary study of narrative therapy for people with chronic pain, *Diversity in Health and Care*, 7, 43–56.

Bury, M. (2001) Illness narratives: fact or fiction? *Sociology of Health & Illness*, 23 (3), 263–285.

de Raeve, L. (2002) The modification of emotional responses: a problem for trust in nurse–patient relationships? *Nursing Ethics*, 9, 465–471.

Fosbinder, D. (1994) Patient perceptions of nursing care: an emerging theory of interpersonal competence, *Journal of Advanced Nursing*, 20, 1085–1093.

Frank, A. (1995) *The Wounded Storyteller: Body, Illness, and Ethics*. Chicago, IL: University of Chicago Press.

Gaydos, H. (2005) Understanding personal narratives: an approach to practice, *Journal of Advanced Nursing*, 49 (3), 254–259.

Gysels, M., Richardson, A. and Higginson, I. (2004) Communication training for health professionals who care for patients with cancer: a systematic review of effectiveness, *Journal of Supportive Care in Cancer*, 12 (10), 692–700.

Jackson, D., Firtko, A. and Edenborough, M. (2007) Personal resilience as a strategy for surviving and thriving in the face of workplace adversity: a literature review, *Journal of Advanced Nursing*, 60 (1), 1–9.

Jarrett, N. and Payne, S. (1995) A selective review of the literature on nurse–patient communication: has the patient's contribution been neglected? *Journal of Advanced Nursing*, 22, 72–78.

Kasch, C. (1986) Towards a theory of nursing action: skills and competency in nurse–patient interaction, *Nursing Research*, 35 (4), 226–229.

Kirk, T. (2007) Beyond empathy: clinical intimacy in nursing practice, *Nursing Philosophy*, 8, 233–243.

Kitson, A. (1993) Formalizing concepts relating to nursing and caring, in Kitson, A. (ed.) *Nursing: Art and Science*. London: Chapman & Hall.

Macleod Clark, J. (1983) Nurse–patient communication - an analysis of conversations from surgical wards, in Wilson-Barnett, J. (ed.) *Nursing Research: Ten Studies in Patient Care*. Chichester: John Wiley & Sons, pp. 25–56.

May, C. (1991) Affective neutrality and involvement in nurse–patient relationships: perceptions of appropriate behaviour among nurses in acute medical and surgical wards, *Journal of Advanced Nursing*, 16, 552–558.

McCreaddie, M. and Wiggins, S. (2007) The purpose and function of humour in health, health care and nursing: a narrative review, *Journal of Advanced Nursing*, 61 (6), 584–595.

McMahon, R. (1991) Therapeutic nursing: theory, issues and practice, in McMahon, R. and Pearson, A. (eds) *Nursing as Therapy*. London: Chapman & Hall, pp. 1–25.

Menzies Lyth, I. (1959) The functioning of social systems as a defence against anxiety, in Menzies Lyth, I. (1988) *Containing Anxiety in Institutions: Selected Essays*. London: Free Associated Books, pp. 43–85.

Morse, J. (1991) Negotiating commitment and involvement in the nurse–patient relationship, *Journal of Advanced Nursing*, 16, 455–468.

Noble, A. and Jones, C. (2005) Benefits of narrative therapy: holistic interventions at the end of life, *British Journal of Nursing*, 14 (6), 330–333.

Papstavrou, E., Efstathiou, G., Tsangari, H., Suhonen, R., Leino-Kilpi, H., Patiraki, E., Karlou, C., Balogh, Z., Palese, A., Tomietto, M., Jarosova, D. and Merkouris, A. (2011) A cross-cultural study of the concept of caring through behaviours: patients' and nurses' perspectives in six different EU countries, *Journal of Advanced Nursing*, 68 (5), 1026–1037.

Peplau, H. (1969) Professional closeness, *Nursing Forum*, 8 (4), 342–360.

Peplau, H. (1972) *Interpersonal Relations in Nursing*. Basingstoke: Macmillan Education.

Ramos, M. (1992) The nurse–patient relationship: theme and variations, *Journal of Advanced Nursing*, 17, 496–506.

Roberts, D. and Snowball, J. (1999) Psychosocial care in oncology nursing: a study of social knowledge, *Journal of Clinical Nursing*, 8, 39–47.

Savage, J. (1995) *Nursing Intimacy*. London: Scutari Press.

Severinsson, E. (2001) Confirmation, meaning and self-awareness as core concepts of the nursing supervision model, *Nursing Ethics*, 8 (1), 36–44.

Smith, P. (1992) *The Emotional Labour of Nursing*. Basingstoke: Macmillan.

Thomas-MacLean, R. (2004) Understanding breast cancer stories via Frank's narrative types, *Social Science & Medicine*, 58 (9), 1647–1657.

Webster, M. (1981) Communication with dying patients, *Nursing Times*, 77, 999–1002.

Williams, A. (2001) A literature review on the concept of intimacy in nursing, *Journal of Advanced Nursing*, 33 (5), 660–667.

Williams, A. and Irurita, V. (2004) Therapeutic and non-therapeutic interpersonal interactions: the patient's perspective, *Journal of Clinical Nursing*, 13, 806–815.

Williams, G. (1984) The genesis of chronic illness: narrative re-construction, *Sociology of Health & Illness*, 6 (2), 175–200.

Wiseman, T. (1996) A concept analysis of empathy, *Journal of Advanced Nursing*, 23, 1162–1167.

Further reading

Polkinghorne, D. (1988) *Narrative Knowing and the Human Sciences*. State University of New York Press: Albany, NY.

Schutz, S. and Bulman, C. (2008) *Reflective Practice in Nursing* (4th edition). Oxford: Blackwell.

4

PSYCHOSOCIAL ASSESSMENT
Understanding the Whole Person

Learning outcomes

By the end of this chapter, you should be able to:

- understand the purpose of psychosocial assessment within the context of a holistic approach to nursing care;
- recognize different dimensions of assessment and how to integrate them into care planning;
- analyse the meaning of patients' own accounts of their condition;
- develop the skills to undertake effective assessment based on a comprehensive evaluation of the patient's condition.

Introduction

A holistic approach to assessment is a key element of psychosocial nursing care. This needs to take account of a range of dimensions of the patient's life. As an interaction between patient and nurse, the assessment also has the potential to be therapeutic for the patient by enabling them to tell their own story of health and illness in their own terms. A psychosocial assessment is one that takes account of physical, psychological, social and spiritual aspects of the patient's life in a balanced and integrated way, achieving an assessment of the whole person.

The purpose of psychosocial assessment

The primary purpose of psychosocial assessment is to collect information that will enable the nurse to plan and deliver effective nursing care, often as part of an inter-professional or multidisciplinary treatment plan. It also has other functions:

- It is part of the process of engagement and collaboration with the patient.
- It provides an opportunity for dialogue and for the patient to ask questions.

- It can provide the nurse with a deeper understanding of the nature of the patient's experience of health and illness.
- It can have therapeutic benefits for the patient, by enabling them to reflect on their experience of illness and construct a personal narrative.

The specific purpose of an assessment will vary according to the circumstances. Assessment may be a single event but it is often part of a process of care over time, and the emphasis will vary according to care and treatment priorities and the patient's condition. Box 4.1 shows common elements for assessment of a patient. If we consider a particular patient as an example: you are working with a patient who has been recently diagnosed with insulin-dependent diabetes, your priority would be to identify how effectively the patient is managing their condition, so the questions below would help to identify the underlying personal and emotional processes.

Box 4.1 Different elements of psychosocial assessment

- Identify how the patient is responding to their health problems (e.g. do they have a positive attitude to the management of their diabetes or are they feeling it is too much for them to cope with?)
- Elicit concerns and sources of personal distress (e.g. what are they mainly concerned about at the moment: the diabetes, or are there other things on their mind?)
- Understand the patient's current social circumstances (e.g. how are their most important relationships being affected by their new circumstances?)
- Screen for the presence of mental illness and other risk factors (e.g. has there been a change in their mood recently, and is this having an impact on how they manage the diabetes?)
- Identify sources of support and personal meaning for the patient (e.g. does the patient have support from family and friends, and any other personal important sources of social, psychological or spiritual support?)

Narrative as a basis for assessment

Assessment as a process represents a balance between two major factors: what the nurse needs to know and what the patient wants and is able to tell them. The nurse will be motivated by their professional background and training to focus on particular aspects of the patient's condition. They will also be strongly influenced by the nature of their role and the speciality within which they are employed. There will be things that they need to know in order to plan care effectively.

At a basic level, the patient can communicate with the nurse as a simple sharing of information. However, the patient will have their own sense of their needs and priorities, and how these fit within their view of their health and illness and other aspects of their life. As we saw in Chapter 2, the way they communicate this more complex picture can be understood as a form of *narrative*. A narrative has the following characteristics: it describes a number of events (i.e. at least two), and it describes causal relationships. A story is a form of narrative that also provides detail of a problematic issue, with an explanation related to it, the characters involved, and it has an emotional effect (Paley and Eva 2005). Box 4.2 gives examples of these different forms of information-sharing and narrative.

A narrative therefore gives more personal detail than a simple exchange of information, and has the potential to represent the emotional quality of a patient's experience and give *personal meaning* to their account. The simple narrative given as an

Box 4.2 Types of narrative (based on Paley and Eva 2005)

	Qualities	Produces	Example
Information-sharing	Information given and received	Basic information	'I am feeling quite down.'
Narrative	• Events (at least two) • Causal relationships	Detailed information from the patient's perspective	'I am feeling quite down. To be honest, I have been feeling down for the last few weeks since I got my test results. They were quite bad and I fear the worst. I saw Dr Smith three weeks ago, and she bluntly told me that my tumour has not responded to treatment.'
Narrative: story	• A problematic issue • A related explanation • The characters involved • An emotional effect	Detailed information from the patient's perspective, which includes: • Emotional effect • Personal Meaning	'I am feeling quite down. To be honest, I have been feeling down for the last three weeks since I got my test results. They were quite bad and I fear the worst. I saw Dr Smith three weeks ago, and she bluntly told me that my tumour has not responded to treatment. So every time I think of something I was looking forward to – like my 30th wedding anniversary in six months' time – I just think, "Oh what's the point?" There's no hope any more, is there?'

example in Box 4.2 implies a causal connection between events, while the story has a more detailed function. It invites the nurse's sympathy, implies a criticism of the doctor, it tells you something about what is important to the patient (their marriage, their family) and the question at the end suggests that either they have given up hope or that they could be more hopeful if the nurse can give them a reason to be.

Asking questions to gain an understanding of the patient's narrative can be the aim of the assessment, and narrative can be the process by which assessment takes place; that is, *narrative assessment.* This approach to assessment involves asking a limited number of questions, encouraging the patient to tell their own story in their own words.

A narrative form of assessment is important in that it provides an opportunity to explore the ways in which the patient understands their illness. This may involve both medical and *lay terminology* or personal words and meanings. One of the effects of Dualism and medical specialization has been to focus the attention of health care staff on signs and symptoms, and not on the whole person (Bury 2001). Narrative assessment gives an opportunity to see signs and symptoms within a broader personal and social context. In its most simple and basic form, a narrative assessment starts with an open question: *Can you tell me about . . . ?*

Priorities, time and setting

However, in dealing with personal narrative, it is important to understand that there is a distinction between the narrative truth of a person's story and the objective truth of events (Paley and Eva 2005). That is, facts may become reinterpreted, re-emphasized or put in a different order in the construction of a personal narrative. There is a tension between the patient's narrative and the demands of the assessment itself. For this reason, the nurse needs to be analytical in their approach to the information that the patient provides. What is it necessary to know to complete the assessment? What is it important for the patient to say in developing their narrative?

The setting, the time available and the condition of the patient will affect how the interview is conducted and what aims are realistic for the outcomes of the assessment. In situations where there is limited time, clinical priorities are acute, or the patient's physical or mental condition is poor, then a limited assessment, focused on information-sharing alone, may be the only option. In most cases a narrative account is preferable, as it provides links between events and causes. This enables a symptom to be understood within the personal context of the individual. Where more time is available, then it is possible to explore personal feelings and meanings in more detail (see the examples in Box 4.2). Like any form of communication, assessment should ideally take place in a private area free of interruptions. Where this is not possible, every attempt should be made to provide private space that will give the patient a sense of trust in the confidentiality of the assessment process.

The process of assessment

The interpersonal process of assessment is based on the communication skills outlined in Chapter 2 and the relationship skills in Chapter 3. The key elements of the process are as follows.

Observing

Much of communication is non-verbal. Observation is the key to understanding the non-verbal cues given by the patient, and also to interpreting their presentation (see Box 4.3). Presentation means the general demeanour of the patient, their posture, position, dress, and any other signs that give a picture of the patient's mood, energy and health. This information is complementary to the verbal information given by the patient.

Box 4.3 Non-verbal cues and signs

Posture – slumped or alert

Position – turned towards or away from the nurse

Eye contact – engaged, withdrawn, distracted, warm

Facial expression – e.g. smiling, blank, tense, worried, angry

Hand gestures – these require energy so may be absent when fatigued

Behaviour – e.g. agitated, restless, disengaged, tearful

Eliciting and gathering information

This is mainly a verbal process, involving asking questions and listening.

Clarifying and responding

It is important to establish that there are mutual understandings of the information shared. The patient also needs to know what will be done with the information that they have provided to the nurse. See Box 4.4 for the process of gathering information and responding to the patient. See also Chapter 2, Boxes 7, 8 and 9 for examples of questioning and responding.

Box 4.4 Verbal process of assessment

1. Introduction of people present and purpose of assessment
2. Asking questions
3. Listening, clarifying and responding
4. Checking for understanding
5. Inviting questions
6. Summarizing and closing

Dimensions of assessment

Within an integrated or holistic approach, care needs to be taken in how any symptoms are interpreted. *Presenting problems* do not always give an immediate guide to the underlying problem (see discussion of medically unexplained physical symptoms in Chapter 1, p. 14). For example, the majority of people who are depressed report physical, not psychological, symptoms (see Chapter 7). On the other hand, a general statement of distress may hide specific physical or psychological symptoms. This underlines the importance of holistic assessment, considering all elements of a patient's experience of health together.

Physical assessment

Function and activity

Changes to physical functioning represent a change from what is experienced as normal by the patient. Traditional approaches to rehabilitation have emphasized a return to 'normal', though this implies full recovery of previous function, which is not always possible. In life-threatening illness, the aim may be to achieve a 'new normal', which represents changes as a result of the process of illness and treatment, including both positives and negatives (Doyle 2008). What a patient is able to do, and the discrepancy between what they want to do and what they can actually do, are essential elements of physical assessment. It is also important to establish how they are adjusting to any limitations on their function, either temporary or permanent.

Case study (Tracey Brown from Chapter 1)

The nurse working with Tracey can move beyond the physical assessment of her function and mobility to assess the impact of the injuries on her life and the meanings attached to function and activity. The following examples are generic questions that could be used with any patient. Thinking specifically about this case, they also show how the nurse could frame her questions to explore the wider impact of the injuries on Tracey's life.

Key questions

1. Do you have any limitations on your function as a result of the illness or treatment (or accident)?
2. Do you feel frustrated by any of the things that you want to do but can't?
3. Have you been able to make adjustments to what you can't do as a result of the illness?
4. Is there anything that you need support to do?

Sleep

Sleep has a restorative function for the body, the mind and the emotions, and is a vital part of physical and mental health. A lack of good quality sleep leads not only to tiredness, but also to poor attention and memory, disorientation, irritability and low mood (Espie 2010). Sleep disturbance is associated with many psychological health problems, including depression (see Chapter 7). *Sleep hygiene*, which is establishing a healthy lifestyle and preparation for sleep, is something that can be introduced to anyone experiencing problems with sleep. This can include advice on exercise, diet and the sleep environment and how these impact on sleep (Espie 2010). Insomnia and other sleep problems can also be helped using cognitive behavioural techniques.

Key questions

- Do you have problems getting off to sleep?
- When do you wake up? Is this the usual time for you?
- Is your sleep pattern broken?
- Do you find your sleep satisfying and refreshing?
- Are you taking anything to help you sleep?

Appetite and diet

Appetite disturbance is a feature of many physical and psychological problems (see Chapters 6 and 7). Eating has a social, cultural, emotional and, for some, a spiritual or religious function, as well as physiological function, so disruption of normal eating patterns (e.g. after surgery of the head and neck) can have an impact on social relationships and personal identity. The eating disorders *anorexia nervosa* and *bulimia nervosa* are psychiatric conditions that can be associated with other disorders of mood and control, for example depression and, drug misuse. Loss of appetite is more serious if associated with significant weight loss.

Key questions

- Do you enjoy your food?
- Have you lost weight? How much and over what period?
- Do you have any problems eating with family and friends?
- Does your diet have any special meaning for you?

Case study (Andy Clarke from Chapter 1)

Andy has to change his diet as a result of a recent diagnosis of diabetes. For him, this could have a negative impact on his sense of personal and social identity. Which questions would you ask him to explore what this impact could be and how it could be overcome?

Gastrointestinal disturbances

Gastrointestinal disturbances are often linked to the patient's emotional state, and this is also represented in lay perceptions; for example, *having a gut feeling*. Constipation is common in depression and can be its presenting feature, and diarrhoea is often a feature of anxiety. There are several gastrointestinal disturbances that are classified as *functional gastrointestinal disorders*; that is, persistent and recurring gastrointestinal symptoms that are not caused by tumours or biochemical abnormalities. These include irritable bowel syndrome (IBS), functional heartburn, dyspepsia, and dysphagia, functional constipation and rectal pain. They are commonly associated with reduced quality of life and comorbid psychological disorders (Levy et al 2006).

IBS is a relatively common condition that presents primarily with abdominal discomfort, associated with diarrhoea, constipation, alternations between the two or pain. There are often feelings of urgency, bloating and abdominal distension. It is commonly comorbid with anxiety and depression, and there has been considerable debate about whether these conditions precede diagnosis or are the result of IBS (Sykes et al 2003).

Key questions

- Have you found anything that you do that improves your symptoms?
- What effects are your health problems having on your day-to-day life?

Fatigue

Fatigue is a feature of many physical and psychological disorders, and is a common presentation in primary care. Persistent and long-lasting fatigue that is not relieved by rest, *chronic fatigue*, is a distressing feature of many conditions, including blood disorders, metabolic disturbances, endocrine disorders, heart disease, neurological disorders, infectious diseases, sleep disorders, gastrointestinal and eating disorders, drug and alcohol misuse, depression, and cancer and its treatments.

Chronic fatigue syndrome (CFS), also known as myalgic encephalomyelitis or post-viral fatigue, is a debilitating condition that usually appears first after a viral illness. Its primary feature is severe tiredness and exhaustion. Other symptoms can include malaise after exercise, muscle and joint pain, sore throat and headaches, night sweats and unrefreshing sleep. Cognitive problems, including poor attention, concentration and memory, are common, and CFS is frequently comorbid with depression (Afari and Buchwald 2003).

Although there are clearly both physical and psychological features of the condition, no satisfactory aetiology has yet been established. Viruses, genetic factors, neurological abnormalities, psychiatric disorders and coping style have all been explored as possible causative factors (Afari and Buchwald 2003). Whatever the causes of CFS, though, it can be helped with psychological treatments. A major trial has suggested that CFS responds well to cognitive behavioural therapy (CBT) and graded exercise therapy (White et al 2011). CFS is a very good example of the complexity of conditions that have overlapping psychological, social and physical implications. There remain major controversies among both doctors and patient groups over what the condition should be called, the effectiveness of treatments, and whether research funding should target physiological or psychological treatments (Wikipedia 2012).

The management of fatigue includes addressing and treating the causes, where these can be identified. Additional factors to consider are: balancing rest and exercise; pacing and prioritizing; adequate hydration and nutrition; and sleep hygiene.

Key questions

- Does your fatigue get better after you rest?
- Are you able to take any exercise?
- Is there anything that you do that helps you to relax?
- What effects is fatigue having on your life?

Pain

Pain is a universal human experience and one of the most common reasons for seeking health care. Complaints of pain indicate that something is wrong and in most cases a physical explanation can be found and acted on. The cause of the pain can then be dealt with, or pain management strategies can be initiated. This is the usual course of *acute pain*.

However, pain is not solely a physical sensation. It is an experience that crosses physical, psychological and spiritual boundaries. For example, we can talk about mental pain, spiritual pain and existential pain. Pain is an intrinsically subjective and emotional experience, and this becomes more apparent during the course of *chronic pain*, that is, pain lasting longer than three months. Chronic pain poses particular challenges in practice, as it does not respond to treatments in the ways that would be expected. There has been considerable interest therefore in psychological aspects of its causation, maintenance and how it can be managed. Chronic pain is associated with anxiety, depression, sleep disorders, drug and alcohol misuse, social and relationship problems and suicide (Lumley et al 2011).

The mechanisms underlying pain are extremely complex and involve different neurological pathways. People experience painful stimuli in different ways, and we know that there are a number of personal factors that influence how pain is felt, interpreted and reported. Some of the factors that influence the experience of pain are the individual coping style, the appraisal of the nature of the pain, and what the pain is attributed to, that is, beliefs about the causes of pain (Lumley et al 2011). A tendency to *catastrophization* (see Chapter 6) is also strongly associated with the experience of chronic pain (Quartana et al 2009). The assessment of pain can be very specific to the patient, their condition and the circumstances. However, the following questions will help to get a better understanding of the personal experience of pain.

Key questions

- What does your pain feel like?
- What words would you use to describe the pain?

- What do you think is the cause of your pain?
- What do you think would help you to cope with your pain right now?

Psychological assessment

Thoughts and feelings

The patient's psychological state is mainly assessed by their reports of their thoughts and feelings. Together, these can be termed *cognitions*, and this term is used extensively in *cognitive behavioural therapy (CBT)* (see Chapter 5). Thoughts are ideas or beliefs, usually experienced in words, though sometimes also as mental images. Thoughts are largely consciously experienced, though it is possible to identify thoughts that are not fully conscious (i.e. just below the level of consciousness). Feelings are emotional experiences, and they can usually be summed up in one word; for example, sad, angry, anxious, happy. In contrast, thoughts can have more complex forms as they involve elements of meaning and belief about the self, others or the world (see Box 4.5).

Box 4.5 Thoughts and feelings			
Thought:	'I am a failure'	Feeling:	sad
Thought:	'what happened to me is unfair'	Feeling:	angry
Thought:	'I am going to die'	Feeling:	anxious
Thought:	'the world is a beautiful place'	Feeling:	happy

Thoughts and feelings can both be used to identify a person's *mood*. The feeling encapsulates the mood, for example anxious, depressed, but thoughts can identify the meanings and beliefs that underlie the mood, and they provide the primary focus for most CBT interventions (see Chapter 5). As a general principle, the *ventilation of feelings* within a supportive professional relationship is helpful for people who have experienced stress or trauma or are going through a period of adjustment, though it may not be enough on its own to enable positive growth.

Key questions

- How are you feeling today?
- How would you describe your mood?
- Do you have any particular thoughts that are troubling you?
- What is on your mind?

Mood

The most common psychological problems are the mood disorders anxiety and depression. The assessment of mood is therefore a key element of psychosocial assessment. Mood may be positive or negative. Good mood is associated with happiness or contentment, which are very subjective and personal experiences. Mood problems are also sometimes described as *distress*, and this can have a general meaning of suffering (e.g. symptom distress), discontent or unhappiness, or more specifically refer to the presence of a mental health problem. 'Distress' can also be used slightly differently to describe being upset or tearful, in contrast to more severe psychological problems. For further details of the assessment of mood, see Chapters 6 and 7.

Behaviour

Psychosocial assessment should include assessment of behaviour, the things that people do in response to problems. Behavioural responses to illness can show evidence of anxiety: agitation, restlessness or depression: retardation or slowing up. Behaviour may be an expression of *emotion-focused coping*, for example seeking reassurance, confiding in friends, or *problem-focused coping*, including seeking information, making plans to deal with change. Behaviour may also be *avoidant*, that is, avoiding problems by ignoring or denying them, or finding escape in alcohol or drugs.

Cognitive function

In addition to the concept of cognition as thoughts and feelings, *cognitive* also refers to the mental capacity for concentration, attention and memory. Mild cognitive dysfunction may be associated with anxiety and stress, but more severe dysfunction is usually caused by trauma, psychosis or organic changes. Assessment of cognitive function is explored in more detail in Chapter 8.

Social identity and relationships

Altered body image and self-esteem

Changes to body image are common in physical illness, often though not always accompanied by functional changes. Altered image can occur after surgery, after radiotherapy and chemotherapy (including hair loss), as a result of drug treatments (e.g. corticosteroids), and with weight gain or weight loss. Altered body image can also occur for psychological reasons: *body dysmorphic disorder* and *eating disorders* are characterized by distorted body image.

Body image is closely linked to *self-esteem:* having a self-image that supports a sense of personal value. Although body image is related to self-image, it is also an important element of social identity. Disturbance of body image can lead to disruptions of social functioning, including problems socializing, loss of dignity and sexual problems. In severe cases, this can lead to *social anxiety* that further inhibits social interaction (Newell 2002).

Key questions

- How do you feel about your personal appearance now?
- Are there any things you have stopped doing because you do not feel comfortable with people?

Sexuality

Sexuality is a feature of human health, and is closely bound up with personal and social identity. Illness frequently affects the experience and function of sexuality. *Sexual dysfunction* can include:

- loss of personal feelings of attractiveness;
- reduced sexual desire or arousal;
- inhibited sexual performance;
- loss of orgasm.

Altered body image, fatigue, pain, anxiety and depression, drug and alcohol misuse can all impact on personal sexuality. Sexual problems are usually experienced within a couple and may benefit from being addressed with both partners. Sexuality is very personal, and is one of the most difficult areas of health to address because of embarrassment talking about it. The *extended PLISSIT model* makes permission-giving the central feature of asking and talking about a patient's sexuality and can therefore be enabling for both nurse and patient (Taylor and Davis 2006). Questions should allow patients to talk or not, as they feel comfortable.

Key questions

- Would you like to talk about this?
- Have you discussed this with your partner?

Occupation and finances

Occupation is a key element of social identity: many people define themselves by what they do, and the workplace is a significant focus of social interaction. Illness commonly disrupts occupational function and can lead to a loss of role, both within the work environment and possibly also at home, if the patient is normally the main wage earner. Illness can place additional financial demands on individuals and families. This can include travel and car parking charges, insurance, new clothing and special diets.

Key questions

- Have you been able to work since being ill?
- Are you in contact with your employer?
- What effects has not working had on you and your family?
- Are you having any financial problems as a result of the illness?

Relationships and social support

Illness can have a number of negative effects on relationships:

- changed family roles (e.g. the sick person may no longer be able to support other family members, or younger members of a family may have to take on roles they do not feel prepared for);
- loss of intimacy;
- loss of an active social life;
- rejection by family or friends who are unable to cope with the illness.

However, illness can also have positive effects on relationships: they can become stronger in the face of adversity, and new relationships can start based on the patient's changed circumstances (e.g. with other people who have the same condition). *Social support* is the term used to describe the supportive elements of relationships, and this can take different forms. It can include companionship and emotional support, information, practical and financial support. In times of ill health, some of this is likely to be provided by health care agencies, and, where the patient's usual social support is not adequate, there may be a role for additional professional support.

Key questions

- Have your relationships changed since your illness?
- How do you feel about this?
- Where do you get your support from?
- Do you feel adequately supported at the moment?

Case study (Andy Clarke from Chapter 1)

In Andy's case, his illness resulted in changes to his social relationships that enabled him to adjust effectively to his condition. If you had concerns about his relationships and support during his adjustment to diabetes, which questions would you ask and how would you decide whether he would benefit from additional support?

The family as a unit of assessment

It is often difficult to understand a person fully outside of the context of their family. However, what constitutes a family varies considerably. In most cases it involves people who are related by blood, though this is not always the case. Families are defined by having a close affiliation on the grounds of blood relationships, living together, or other bonds of friendship or obligation. This is the most common unit of social identity and belonging, where people are nurtured and intimacy is shared. Families may be relatively stable, or they could change frequently, with members being admitted and leaving according to the circumstances. In the case of illness, new members may be admitted to provide extra care, and professionals may be considered effectively members of the family for a limited period. Families are often the unit of care, especially where there is a sick child.

Taking a holistic view of the patient, it is very useful to assess them within the family as a *system*. There are two very useful tools for representing families and relationships in diagrammatic form: genograms and ecomaps. These can aid our understanding of how relationships function, in supporting the patient or making additional demands on them, and seeing how this changes over time.

Genograms

Genograms are a diagrammatic way of representing families. They are very useful for giving a full picture of family history and relationships. They can also be used to plot genetic risk in families where there is a history of inherited illness (see Figure 4.1).

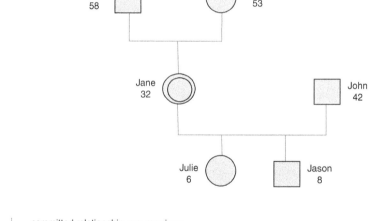

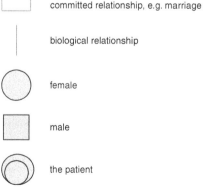

Figure 4.1 Family genogram: the Smith family

Ecomaps

Ecomaps are a visual representation of family units, other social circles or environments that enable social interaction to be explored within the conceptual framework of *systems theory*. They are particularly useful as a tool for analysing relationships. Their flexibility means that they can include any element that you feel is relevant, and they can be redrawn at any point when the characters or the dynamics between them change (see Box 4.6 and Figure 4.2).

Box 4.6 Uses of ecomaps

- Identifying problems within a family or environment
- Planning care and interventions targeting the interface between people
- Identifying where problems are interactional
- Recording a situation or case
- Evaluating outcomes and measuring change

(Hartman 1995)

Case study: the Smith family

Jane Smith has had irritable bowel syndrome for the past five years. She has also been diagnosed with depression and takes antidepressant medication. At times Jane finds it hard to get on with her life, she feels ill and tired, and does not want to get out of bed or go out. She has not had a job since her first child was born eight years ago. Jane does not have a close relationship with her husband, John. He has a demanding job and spends most of his time and energy working. John is not close to his son and daughter, though they get on well, and he sometimes takes them out for social activities when Jane is feeling ill or tired. Jane has a close and loving relationship with her son Jason, but has a difficult relationship with her daughter Julie, with frequent arguments. Julie has had some problems at school. Julie and Jason get on very well together but do not talk about their mother's illness. Jane's parents live nearby and she sees a lot of her father, who is very supportive and sometimes gives her practical help with transport and shopping. She has never got on well with her mother, who does not spend much time with Jane or her family.

Reflection point

- Looking at the ecomap (Figure 4.2), can you identify a professional intervention that would help any specific member of the family?
- Can you identify a point on the ecomap where a change in the relationship between two of the individuals would have a beneficial effect on the whole of the family, and how this might take place?
- Looking at both the genogram and the ecomap, could you a see a use for both or either of them in your practice?

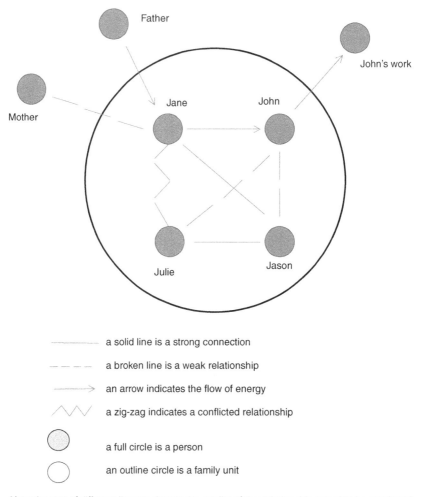

———————	a solid line is a strong connection
– – – –	a broken line is a weak relationship
————→	an arrow indicates the flow of energy
∧∨∨	a zig-zag indicates a conflicted relationship
⬤	a full circle is a person
◯	an outline circle is a family unit

Note: the use of different lines to denote the quality of the relationship can also be employed with genograms.

Figure 4.2 Family ecomap: the Smith family

Exercise

You can do this exercise on your own but it would also be useful to do this with a colleague. Think of a family that you have worked with where you felt there was a problem within the dynamics of the family, or in your relationship with the family. Draw both a genogram and an ecomap of the family. Place yourself on the ecomap, in relation to the family members. Does this help you to see the problem or problems more clearly?

Spiritual assessment

Spirituality is a complex and at times intangible concept, and there is a considerable overlap with other aspects of the individual's personal and social life. Box 4.7 addresses those aspects of the patient's experience that can be judged as spiritual in comparison with those that are psychological or social. It is not always necessary to address the patient's spiritual needs, but these do become prominent if the patient is critically ill or facing death. Spirituality, like sexuality, can be intensely personal and not all patients would want to talk about it within an assessment. Rather, in thinking about spiritual matters, patients value good humour in nurses, and opportunities provided by nurses for quiet time and space (Taylor and Mamier 2005). It is important therefore to provide opportunities for quiet reflection, and to ask questions only if the situation suggests that the patient would welcome the chance to discuss it.

Box 4.7 Spiritual aspects of the patient's experience

- Sense of mortality and existential distress
- Sources of inner energy, strength and hope
- Sense of meaning and purpose in the face of illness
- Transcendence – dimensions of spiritual experience beyond the self
- Religious or philosophical beliefs

The focus of any questions should be to support the patient in their own quest for strength, guidance or meaning.

Key questions

- Would you find it helpful to talk about how you are feeling now?
- Where do you look for your own sense of strength and hope?
- Is there anyone in particular that you feel could help you with these concerns?

Adjustment

In Chapter 1, we saw that people respond to illness with different processes of coping and adjustment, transition and growth. Understanding these processes in an individual will enable the nurse to support them more effectively. Assessing someone's adjustment to their circumstances will include observing their behaviour in response to their illness, or diagnosis, test results etc. The response of the family will also provide information. Important areas for questions can include: coping and appraisal, priorities and goals; personal meanings of events; and opportunities for personal growth and reflection (Box 4.8; see also Chapter 1). It is useful to know what resources are available to the patient that will facilitate their adjustment. The patient may be aware of resources themselves, including both formal and informal sources of support. Giving the patient additional options will then enable them to make choices about how they would like to receive support to aid the process of adjustment.

Case study (Tracey Brown from Chapter 1)

Looking at the questions in Box 4.8, if you were the nurse working with Tracey, which of these questions would you ask her to help her to find ways of adjusting to her injuries?

Box 4.8 Process of adjustment – questions to ask

- What has your previous experience of illness been like, in yourself or others?
- Is there anything more that you would like to know about this condition?
- What has helped you to cope in the past?
- How do you think you will be able to deal with this?
- What are your current priorities in life?
- Do you have any specific goals and do you feel you are able to work towards achieving them at the moment?
- What do you think this (illness/treatment/accident/setback/diagnosis) means for you and your life?
- Have you found any positives in this experience?
- Have you had any chances to reflect on what has been happening to you?
- Would you like to talk about this?
- Have you considered writing this down to help you make sense of what has happened?

Valuing diversity

Valuing diversity in assessment means acknowledging the differences between people, and appreciating the qualities that each person has. As we gain professional experience, we see many people with similar conditions, similar circumstances and similar problems. We all have an inherent tendency to recognize patterns, and this can have the effect of giving us presuppositions about people on the basis of their circumstances. Valuing diversity, on the other hand, is a way of seeing people's unique responses to illness and problems. This is consistent with the models of coping, transition, growth and resilience that were explored in Chapter 1, and using narrative as a means of gaining direct access to personal accounts.

Acknowledging individual difference may not be enough on its own. Differences can also lead to inequalities in access and experience of health care. Factors that can affect this include:

- age
- gender
- sexual orientation
- ethnicity, religion or cultural affiliation
- socioeconomic and employment status
- disability

People who live in poverty have poorer health, more health problems and die younger. People may also experience *social exclusion* because of prejudice or stigma based on their culture or ethnicity. Providing care that responds to cultural diversity may be termed *cultural competence*, and this involves developing cultural self-awareness, and cultural knowledge and cultural skills to meet the needs of a wide range of people (Campinha-Bacote 2002).

Reflection point

Do you have experience of any individual or group of people having problems accessing or using your service? Can you identify what factors contributed to this?

Assessment frameworks and tools

Assessment tools and frameworks can be useful aids to the assessment process. It is important to be clear what the purpose of the tool is. For example, many are designed to be used for research, so would not be suitable for use in day-to-day practice. However, there are a number of tools suitable for use in practice. These are often described under the heading Patient Reported Outcome Measures (PROMS), and are designed to measure patients' perceptions of their general health or their specific health condition as an outcome of care (Dawson et al 2010).

A number of assessment tools that are specific to conditions are described in the following chapters. These include assessment frameworks and screening tools:

Chapter 6 – anxiety

- Distress thermometer
- Hospital Anxiety and Depression Scale (HADS)
- Health Anxiety Inventory (HAI)

Chapter 7 – depression

- Single and double question assessment
- Distress thermometer
- Hospital Anxiety and Depression Scale (HADS)

- Edinburgh Postnatal Depression Scale (EPDS)
- Patient Health Questionnaire (PHQ-9)

Chapter 8 – working with psychosis

Assessment tools

- Mental State Examination
- Mini Mental State Examination (MMSE)
- Confusion Assessment Method (CAM)

Chapter 9 – working with difficult behaviours

Alcohol screening tools

- Alcohol units
- AUDIT
- FAST

Care planning

The outcome of psychosocial assessment should be care that is based a holistic appraisal of the patient's needs. Care can then be planned in *partnership* or *collaboration* with the patient, with an awareness of how it will be understood within the context of the patient's life. Partnership involves an engaged relationship, with the nurse exercising effective interpersonal skills, having self-awareness and being able to negotiate with the patient (Gallant et al 2002).

Summary

Assessment provides the basis for planning and delivering nursing care. Psychosocial assessment offers the potential for developing a deeper understanding of the patient, their problems and their world. The next chapter explores the potential for nurses to go beyond traditional caring roles to more specialized psychological interventions with patients.

Key points

Psychosocial assessment:

- involves a willingness to listen to the patient's account of their symptoms and illness in their own terms;
- addresses physical, psychological, social and spiritual concerns;
- values diversity;
- forms the basis for a partnership in planning and delivering nursing care.

References

Afari, N. and Buchwald, D. (2003) Chronic fatigue syndrome: a review, *American Journal of Psychiatry*, 160 (2), 221–236.

Bury, M. (2001) Illness narratives: fact or fiction? *Sociology of Health & Illness*, 23 (3), 263–285.

Campinha-Bacote, J. (2002) The process of cultural competence in the delivery of healthcare services: a model of care, *Journal of Transcultural Nursing*, 13 (3), 181–184.

Dawson, J., Doll, H., Fitzpatrick, R., Jenkinson, C. and Carr, A. (2010) Routine use of patient reported outcome measures in healthcare settings, *British Medical Journal*, 340, c186.

Doyle, N. (2008) Cancer survivorship: evolutionary concept analysis, *Journal of Advanced Nursing*, 62, 499–509.

Espie, C. (2010) *Overcoming Insomnia and Sleep Problems: A Self-help Guide Using Cognitive Behavioral Techniques*. London: Robinson.

Gallant, M., Beaulieu, M. and Carnevale, F. (2002) Partnership: an analysis of the concept within the nurse–patient relationship, *Journal of Advanced Nursing*, 40 (2), 149–157.

Hartman, A. (1995) Diagrammatic assessment of family relationships, *Families in Society*, 76 (2), 111–122.

Levy, R., Olden, K., Naliboff, B., Bradley, L., Francisconi, C., Drossman, D. and Creed, F. (2006) Psychosocial aspects of functional gastrointestinal disorders, *Gastroenterology*, 130, 1447–1458.

Lumley, M., Cohen, J., Borszcz, G., Cano, A., Radcliffe, A., Porter, L., Schubiner, H. and Keefe, F. (2011) Pain and emotion: a biopsychosocial review of recent research, *Journal of Clinical Psychology*, 67 (9), 942–968.

Newell, R. (2002) Psychological approaches to body image disturbance, in Regel, S. and Roberts, D. (eds) *Mental Health Liaison*. London: Baillière-Tindall.

Paley, J. and Eva, G. (2005) Narrative vigilance: the analysis of stories in health care, *Nursing Philosophy*, 6, 83–97.

Quartana, P., Campbell, C. and Edwards, R. (2009) Pain catastrophizing: a critical review, *Expert Review of Neurotherapeutics*, 9 (5), 745–758.

Sykes, M., Blanchard, E., Lackner, J., Keefer, L. and Krasner, S. (2003) Psychopathology in Irritable Bowel Syndrome: support for a psychophysiological model, *Journal of Behavioral Medicine*, 26 (4), 361–372.

Taylor, B. and Davis, S. (2006) Using the Extended PLISSIT model to address sexual health-care needs, *Nursing Standard*, 21 (11), 35–40.

Taylor, E. and Mamier, I. (2005) Spiritual care nursing: what cancer patients and family care-givers want, *Journal of Advanced Nursing*, 49 (3), 260–267.

White, P., Goldsmith, K., Johnson, A., Walwyn, R., DeCesare, J., Baber, H., Clark, L., Cox, L., Bavington, J., Angus, B., Murphy, G., Murphy, M., O'Dowd, H., Wilks, D., McCrone, P., Chalder, T. and Sharpe, M. (2011) Comparison of adaptive pacing therapy, cognitive behaviour therapy, graded exercise therapy, and specialist medical care for chronic fatigue syndrome (PACE): a randomised trial, *The Lancet*, 377, 823–836.

Wikipedia (2012) Controversies related to chronic fatigue syndrome. Available online at www.en.wikipedia.org/wiki/Controversies_related_to_chronic_fatigue_syndrome (accessed on 19 June 2012).

Wilkinson, R. and Marmot, M. (2003) *Social Determinants of Health: The Solid Facts* (2nd edition), World Health Organization. Available online at www.euro.who.int/en/what-we-publish/abstracts/social-determinants-of-health.-the-solid-facts (accessed on 2 July 2012).

5

PSYCHOTHERAPEUTIC APPROACHES IN NURSING
New Opportunities for Working with the Whole Person

Learning outcomes

By the end of this chapter, you should be able to:

- understand the main psychotherapeutic models and approaches that are relevant to nursing practice;
- recognize elements of counselling and psychotherapy that can be incorporated into nursing;
- explore the potential for developing nursing practice using psychotherapeutic techniques;
- develop effective listening skills in the care of patients and their families.

Introduction

Psychotherapy and nursing have much in common. They both involve close, even intimate, professional working relationships with patients. They both make emotional demands on the professional. They also both have considerable potential to bring about positive change in the lives of people with health problems. However, there are also differences. Psychotherapy is usually theory-driven, structured and systematic. Nursing, in comparison, is often driven by human values, tends to be more reactive to the changing condition of the patient and adaptive to changes in the health care environment. There is, however, much that nursing can learn from psychotherapy, and psychotherapeutic concepts and models have been adapted for use by nurses over a long period of time. This chapter gives an overview of the main counselling and psychotherapy approaches that have potential value for nurses, with a focus on their practical applications.

Counselling and counselling skills

Counselling has enjoyed a popular image among nurses for a very long time. It has also been used as a theoretical basis for understanding nurse–patient communication and relationships, and as a model for specialist nurses relating to their clients. However, it has also been identified that counselling theories, concepts and models do not always fit neatly into the context of nursing care. For example, Bottorff and Morse (1994) argued that a concentration on verbal interactions devalues non-verbal interaction, particularly touch.

Counselling skills can provide a model for understanding and developing the interpersonal verbal aspects of nursing. The basic elements of counselling are *active listening, personal availability of the counsellor* and *the skilled use of questions* to guide a therapeutic interaction. The way that these questions are used is significant. In *non-directive counselling* the counsellor uses questions to aid the client in exploring their emotions according to their own agenda within the interaction (Box 5.1 and also see Chapter 2). In *directive counselling*, the counsellor uses questions to focus on a thera-peutic agenda that fits their perception of the client's problems and their solution. Note: the term *client* is used more commonly than *patient* in counselling and psycho-therapy so will be used throughout this chapter.

Box 5.1 Non-directive counselling skills

- Open and closed questions
- Reflective listening: simple reflection and selective reflection
- Checking for understanding
- Paraphrasing and summaries

Carl Rogers (2004), within his model of client-centred counselling, defined the basic elements of counselling embodied within the counsellor and the therapeutic set-ting. These *core conditions* that are necessary in the counsellor to bring about therapeutic change are empathy, unconditional positive regard and congruence.

- *Empathy* means that the counsellor experiences an accurate, empathic under-standing of the client's experience, and that this is communicated to the client.

- *Unconditional positive regard* refers to the counsellor's acceptance of the client without conditions and without judgement. This enables the client to be more accepting of themselves and their intrinsic value as a person.

- *Congruence* or *genuineness* means that the counsellor gets involved with the client in the therapy sessions in a real and personal way, including sharing their own feelings and responses to the client.

Although Rogers focuses on the interpersonal aspects of the counselling relation-ship, the physical setting is also very important. Effective counselling, based on these core conditions, requires privacy and uninterrupted time. For many nurses, their work setting will not be conducive to developing a counselling relationship. Rogers' counselling model can also be criticized for theoretical reasons. There are limits to how much a professional relationship can be unconditional, given the restrictions placed on it by employers, regulations and codes of conduct, so the full attention of the nurse may be considered an alternative to unconditional positive regard. Genuineness and spontaneity may be difficult to achieve in day-to-day practice, with multiple demands being made on the time and energies of the busy professional, so a respectful and compassionate attitude to the patient may be more realistic. It is important therefore to make a distinction between the use of counselling skills, that is, effective and attentive listening, and careful use of questions, on the one hand, and the practice of counselling, which requires quite specific factors to be present to make it successful, on the other (see Box 5.2).

Box 5.2 Conditions for nurses providing counselling in health settings

- Empathy (in the nurse)
- Unconditional positive regard *or* the full attention and availability of the nurse
- Congruence and genuineness *or* respect and compassion
- Privacy and uninterrupted time
- The nurse has had preparation for the counselling role and has confidence in their skills
- The nurse has a professional understanding of the counselling relationship
- The nurse works within a professional framework and with adequate resources and managerial support
- The nurse has supervision from a suitably qualified counsellor
- The client understands the nature of counselling and is motivated to work towards therapeutic change

---

Motivational interviewing

Motivational interviewing (MI) is a form of directive, client-centred counselling (see Box 5.3). It has a focus on *exploring and resolving ambivalence*; that is, working with the fluctuations in people's readiness to change. It originated in work with people who have problems of alcohol misuse, but now has applications in a range of health problems, including drug misuse, smoking cessation, eating disorders, diabetes management, adherence with psychiatric treatment and health promotion (Britt et al 2004).

Box 5.3 Motivational interviewing: basic principles

- Express empathy
- Develop discrepancy (between personal goals and present behaviour)
- Avoid argument or persuasion
- Roll with resistance
- Support self-efficacy

The counselling style is quiet and facilitative, but directive in helping the client to examine and resolve ambivalence. The motivation must come from the client, and the therapeutic relationship takes the form of a partnership, using interaction to support the client through fluctuations in their readiness to change. Shared activities such as agenda-setting give the client a sense of personal control, but this is balanced by the therapist's use of questions to keep focused on change and the motivation for change. For example, asking questions about drinking might take the following form:

- Tell me some words that describe your positive points as a person.
- Now tell me some words that describe you as a person who has been drinking.
- How do these fit together?

(Britt et al 2004)

You can see from the questions that the therapist is aiming to create a discrepancy between the client's view of themselves and how they are currently behaving. The use of descriptive words rather than sentences keeps the interaction focused and direct. The initiative is then with the client, and the therapist can support and affirm the positive qualities identified by them. Additional techniques are given Box 5.4. Motivational interviewing has great potential for engaging patients in a positive process of change and rewarding nurses with real achievements on the part of patients.

Box 5.4 Motivational interviewing techniques

- Reflective listening
- Expressing acceptance
- Affirmations – statements of recognition about client strengths
- Selective reinforcement of positive motivation
- Monitoring readiness to change
- Affirming self-determination

(Miller and Rollnik 2002)

Psychodynamic psychotherapy

Psychodynamic or psychoanalytic psychotherapies are built on theories that explain human behaviour as being based on unconscious drives and motives. The individual personality evolves in relation to these drives and in response to events and relationships; for example, with parents over the developmental period of childhood and into adulthood. Psychological problems result from unresolved conflicts or tensions arising from the unconscious. For example, the individual may protect the integrity of the personality from difficult unconscious emotions by the denial or repression of feelings.

The practice of individual psychodynamic psychotherapy classically involves the therapist presenting themselves as a 'blank page' on which the patient can present their inner conflicts, and raising the unconscious to the level of consciousness. In this way links can be made between past and present, repressed emotions can be expressed, with the potential for resolution through dialogue with the therapist.

Psychodynamic psychotherapies, and psychoanalysis in general, have become controversial for a number of reasons. They are based on very complex and debatable theory, evidence for their effectiveness is limited and hard to establish, they require intensive training and supervision, and they can be very time-consuming and expensive (for a detailed discussion and critique, see Dryden and Feltham 1992). For these reasons, they have limited applicability within the context of nursing practice. However, they are important because psychodynamic theory has been a factor in the development of nursing, and because some psychodynamic concepts are useful to the practice of nursing. Attachment theory, and two specific concepts, transference and containment, are worthy of further exploration.

Attachment theory

Attachment theory was developed by John Bowlby, based on his work on maternal separation (Holmes 1993). He hypothesized that children become 'attached' to figures who are responsive to them and provide them with consistent care, usually, but not exclusively, parents. This leads to the development of 'internal working models' that guide feelings and expectations in later relationships. Bowlby described *attachment styles*, including secure, where the parent is attentive and responsive, and the child can cope with separation, and insecure styles such as avoidant and ambivalent, where the relationship with the parent is characterized by anxiety and the anticipation of rejection. Avoidant in this context means the child minimizes their needs and keeps the parent at arm's length, and ambivalence, where their reaction may be clinging and submissive, or compensating by providing care for the parent. These patterns then continue into intimate relationships in adult life. Attachment theory has value in nursing as a means of understanding parent–child relationships, and for its role in working with bereavement. It is also a means of explaining difficult nurse–patient relationships where the patient may react to care with avoidance or an uncomfortable level of dependence.

Transference

Transference is used to describe the way that feelings developed during early attachments are transferred onto people with whom we form close relationships at a later point in life. This can include friends, partners, therapists or nurses. Transference feelings are one of the features of the unconscious that can be worked on within dynamic psychotherapy. The key point is that the characteristics of the earlier attachment are transferred, no matter how appropriate they are to the new relationship. Transference feelings may be quite intense (e.g. love or hate) in ways that present difficulties in the nurse–patient relationship. Correspondingly, feelings evoked in the therapist, or nurse, can be equally intense, and this is termed *countertransference*. Both transference and countertransference can be surprising and uncomfortable, evoking feelings quite out of proportion to the situation. Understanding the nature of this phenomenon is the key to resolving it (Jones 2005).

Containment

Containment is a concept from dynamic psychotherapy that refers to when a person's feelings 'spill out' in a way that they cannot control or contain emotionally. At these times people may seek someone to contain what they find uncontainable. In psychotherapy, and in nursing, when these situations arise they are very challenging, and will be experienced as very taxing to the therapist or nurse. However, if the nurse (or therapist) is able to manage themselves, and *hold* the person in an emotional sense, then it provides the patient with a degree of security that allows them to overcome their fear or anxiety. It also provides a model to them of how intense feelings can be contained. Containment is a very useful concept for nurses working with intensely anxious or frightened patients. It is fundamentally different from reassurance, as it provides a sense that *the nurse understands how the patient is feeling*, and can deal with it. Casement (1985) provides examples of how containment works in psychotherapy practice and how it is different from reassurance.

For further examples of the uses of psychodynamic theory in nursing see de Raeve et al (2009) and Barnes et al (1998).

Cognitive therapy

Cognitive therapy, or cognitive behavioural therapy (CBT), is a short-term, structured and focused, collaborative approach to achieving change in the lives of people with psychological problems. It addresses both *cognitive factors*, thoughts, feelings, images and beliefs, and *behavioural factors*, what people do and what meaning they attach to their actions. Unlike psychodynamic therapies, it does not address unconscious processes, but works with conscious cognitive processes to achieve change and to identify underlying belief structures. It is empirical in that it encourages the client to examine the evidence for their beliefs and attitudes towards the world and their problems, and it uses *Socratic questioning* or *guided discovery* as a means of encouraging this. Socratic questioning encourages the client to discover their own answers to questions as a process of learning about their life, its problems and solutions (Box 5.5).

Box 5.5 Examples of Socratic questions

Your client believes that people avoid speaking to them at social events.

- What makes you believe that?
- Can you give me any evidence to support your belief?
- Can you think of any times when this did not happen?
- Is there a different way that you could see this?
- If a friend of yours thought that, what would you say to them?
- What would happen if you made the first move, and spoke to someone else at a social event?

Also, keeping diaries of cognitions (thoughts and feelings) helps to identify *negative automatic thoughts* and to challenge them by, for example, *examining evidence for and against* them, or conducting a *behavioural experiment*. Behavioural experiments are conducted by the patient making a prediction, based on their assumptions, on the outcome of an action, which is then tested out. For example, someone who believes they are not worth getting to know may avoid people to prevent being rejected. However, an experiment in talking to people at a social event may provide evidence that others are interested in talking to them. Discovering the meaning attached to thoughts, feelings and events is important as this enables understanding of the underlying belief structures (assumptions about the world, and core beliefs or schema) that lead to people having psychological problems. Working with cognitions and changing them has an impact on the underlying core beliefs, and it is also possible to work directly with core beliefs through schema-focused CBT (see Box 5.6).

Box 5.6 CBT basic concepts

- Cognitions (thoughts, feelings, mental images)
- Behaviour (what we do and say)
- Negative automatic thoughts (habitual thinking responses to situations that represent underlying beliefs, e.g. 'people think I am an idiot')
- Assumptions or rules for living (usually 'if...then...' statements, e.g. 'If I am not the best at everything then I am useless')
- Core beliefs (e.g. 'I am useless')

Like counselling, CBT requires certain basic qualities in the therapist: warmth, genuineness and accurate empathy (Beck et al 1979). However, unlike counselling, these are believed to be insufficient to bring about therapeutic change. Rather, a structured, systematic approach is needed. This involves processes of setting goals for therapy and agendas for therapy sessions, specific tasks outside of the therapy sessions (sometimes called homework), self-monitoring (e.g. diaries), measurements of mood and regular review (see Box 5.7). Guiding therapy is an individual *formulation* or conceptualization, a model of the person's problems and their origins, using the CBT concepts outlined in Box 5.6. Figure 5.1 gives a simple example of a formulation.

Box 5.7 Process of CBT

- Introduction to the model
- Goal-setting
- Agenda-setting
- Tasks – homework and review
- Self-monitoring and measurement
- Formulation

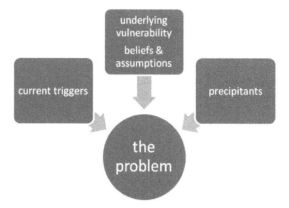

Figure 5.1 Basic CBT formulation

CBT treatment strategies

Treatment strategies in CBT involve both cognitive and behavioural approaches, and it is common to use a combination of both (see Box 5.8). Recording thoughts and feelings in a diary is a common way to initiate the process of change, as it provides a focus for the appraisal and challenge of thoughts or for behavioural experiments (see Figure 5.2, which shows excerpts from a diary of positive events). Mood can be rated or measured as a means of monitoring progress. Behavioural strategies like relaxation and exercise reduce anxiety and activity scheduling enhances the patient's sense of personal control (see Chapter 7, Figure 7.1). The goal of treatment is to achieve a new, more balanced approach to life that enables problems to be overcome and promotes more effective coping.

Box 5.8 CBT treatment strategies

Cognitive

- Identifying cognitions (diary-keeping)
- Appraising and testing automatic thoughts and images
- Developing new perspectives

Behavioural

- Relaxation
- Controlled breathing
- Physical exercise
- Activity scheduling
- Behavioural experiments

Day	Event	What it says about me & my life
Friday	My partner cuddled up to me and told me he loved me	He still loves me in spite of the cancer.
Saturday	I went to a party with my partner and saw friends. They were pleased to see me and liked my wig. Had a good time.	We do normal things. My life is not dominated by cancer.
Sunday	Sister phoned me. Had a chat about Mum and what a terrible time she went through with her cancer.	I was a bit upset but we both agreed she had a much worse time than me. Treatments are so much better these days.
Monday	I had a hospital appointment – good news, I am responding well to treatment.	Not everything is bad news in hospital.

Figure 5.2. Excerpt from Gemma Turner's diary (see case study in Chapter 1, p. 11)

CBT treatment manuals are a means of defining and standardizing treatment. Some of these can be used by patients with or without a therapist, and may also be used in research as the basis for the evaluation of treatment. Box 5.9 gives a summary of one manual-based CBT approach. Given the relatively straightforward nature of some CBT techniques, they are amenable to use by patients themselves as a form of individual self-help based on CBT principles. This includes computerized cognitive behavioural therapy (CCBT) (www.guidance.nice.org.uk/TA97). There is clear evidence for the effectiveness of CBT in the following disorders: depression, generalized anxiety disorder, panic, phobias, obsessive compulsive disorder, post-traumatic stress disorder and bulimia (Roth and Fonagy 2005).

Box 5.9 An example of manual-based CBT

- Identify the problems
- Identify and rate moods
- Thought and mood records
- Identify automatic thoughts
- Seek evidence for and against
- Conduct behavioural experiments
- Find alternatives and develop more balanced thinking

(Greenberger and Padesky 1995)

Problem-solving

Problem-solving therapy (PST) is a CBT technique that has been proven to be effective with a range of disorders, including depression, and can be effectively carried out by nurses after training. It is collaborative, in that the nurse helps the patient to identify problems and generate solutions, with the aim that the patient gains a greater sense of control over their life. As a process it involves the nurse and patient sitting down, the patient with a notebook, and working through a series of steps (see Box 5.10).

Box 5.10 Problem-solving: steps

1.   Identify and define the problem(s)
2.   Brainstorm solution option(s)
3.   Decide which option(s) are achievable
4.   Choose the most feasible option(s)
5.   Prepare and plan strategies to accomplish solution
6.   Try out, evaluate, review

PST enhances the sense of personal control in life and is very helpful in people who are depressed, or for people who are going through difficult life circumstances that feel like they are out of their control.

Case study: Problem-solving treatment

This is a continuation of the case involving Mrs Patel from Chapter 1. Following her meeting with the practice nurse, Mrs Patel sees her general practitioner (GP). Her GP feels she does have features of depression but that also there seem to be underlying problems that it would be helpful for her to talk about. She suggests making a referral to the practice counsellor, aware that Mrs Patel had expressed reluctance to see her. The GP describes the counsellor as an older professional woman with training in specific psychotherapy techniques. She also reinforces the confidential nature of the therapy. Mrs Patel agrees to meet her, if it would help.

Helen Flowers worked as a nurse before training as a counsellor and she has also had additional training in CBT. On assessing Mrs Patel, she decides to take a problem-solving approach. She feels this is suitable for her mild depressed mood, and she also feels it will be empowering for her. The first meeting is an assessment of Mrs Patel's problems, developing rapport and introducing the problem-solving approach. At subsequent meetings, they work together to develop a problem list. This includes her aches and pains and how they make her feel tired, finding it hard to do the housework and keep up with her children's school and other commitments, missing her family who live a long way away, and feeling that her husband is not sympathetic. Brainstorming solutions, she feels talking to her husband about her loneliness, and travelling to her family more would be ideal solutions, but she does not feel these are achievable. Mrs Patel has some ideas about feeling better about herself and her role with the house and with the children, and, in collaboration with Helen, chooses to try and exercise more regularly, initially taking walks with her children, especially when it is to and from their school and other activities, instead of taking the car as she had done previously. She also plans her housework and does it in small doses so she does not feel overwhelmed by it.

Over the next few weeks, she gradually builds her confidence, and says she is beginning to enjoy her time more with her children and feel more on top of things. She is eating a better diet. Reviewing her progress, Helen spends time listening to her remaining concerns, affirming her feelings and supporting her in planning the next steps. Mrs Patel decides she would like to talk to her husband about how she is missing her family, and whether they could arrange a trip to see them. Helen notices a change in the topics she brings up in their sessions. She mentions her aches and pains less as time goes on. Helen has decided not to discuss them directly in her conversations with Mrs Patel, but to focus on how she is feeling generally, about herself and about her life.

Mindfulness

Mindfulness is a meditation technique based in Buddhist principles. It can be summarized as directly experiencing mental and physical processes: thoughts, images, feelings, and sensations, and external stimuli in a non-judgemental way as they arise in the mind. Thoughts and feelings are neither pushed away nor held onto, through mindfulness practice, they are simply experienced. There are two main forms of mindfulness-based psychotherapy: Mindfulness-based cognitive therapy (MBCT) and mindfulness-based stress reduction (MBSR). MBSR has been used with beneficial effects in people with chronic pain and other long-term conditions, and MBCT has demonstrated effectiveness in reducing relapse in people with major depression (Baer 2003). The basic principles of mindfulness therapies are fairly straightforward, and groups based on this approach could be run by nurses with some training.

Links

Mindfulness-based cognitive therapy (MBCT): www.mbct.co.uk/

Mindfulness-based stress reduction (MBSR): www.mindfullivingprograms.com/whatMBSR.php

Psychotherapy – what is the potential for its use in adult general nursing?

There is increasing evidence of the benefits and effectiveness of psychotherapy (for a detailed critical review, see Roth and Fonagy 2005). In the United Kingdom, the government initiative *Improving Access to Psychological Therapies* (IAPT – www.iapt.nhs.uk/about-iapt/) has been set up to increase the number of people who can get specialist help for depression and anxiety and other psychological problems that respond to brief CBT-based therapies. However, access remains limited, and it is unlikely that there will be sufficient practising psychotherapists to deal with the scale of psychological problems in the community. As psychological problems like anxiety and depression are widely found in the physically ill, it makes sense to develop nurses as providers of psychological therapies.

There are a number of studies that highlight the potential of nurses to deliver psychotherapeutic interventions. Some of these highlight training alone, and others evaluate training and outcome studies.

Studies of nurses being trained in psychotherapeutic techniques

Palliative care is a setting where psychosocial problems are well recognized and staff generally have a positive attitude to psychosocial aspects of care. Mannix et al's (2006) study involved training palliative care practitioners in a brief form of CBT, which they term *cognitive first aid*. This covers all of the key features of CBT practice, including cognitive models of anxiety, panic and depression, adjusted for use with people who have life-threatening illness. The sample of 20 trainees included 16 nurses. The training programme was nine days of teaching, followed by three months of fortnightly supervision. The trainees were then randomly allocated to two groups: further supervision or no further supervision.

Both groups showed an increase in competence in the use of CBT skills between baseline and the end of the training period. The group without extended supervision showed a decline in competence between 6 and 12 months after training. The group with extended supervision, however, continued to improve, with a statistically significant difference at 12 months. The nurses in this group were also more likely to use specific CBT techniques: modifying automatic thoughts, use of formulation, using the cognitive model of depression and modifying core beliefs. In a similar study reported by Cort et al (2009), 15 palliative care nurses were given basic training in CBT. They reported increased confidence in working with distressed patients, and in gaining greater depth in the therapeutic relationship.

In a study of nurses working with diabetes, Maissi et al (2011) found similar results. They developed a two-day training programme in motivational enhancement therapy (MET), a form of motivational interviewing, and a five-day training in CBT skills. Both programmes were tailored to the needs of people with diabetes. The six participating nurses were also given supervision on their casework with patients. All of the participants were assessed as having satisfactory to high levels of competence on sample recorded sessions from their practice after training.

These training programmes were tailored to the needs of specific patient groups, and the participants were experienced specialist nurses, who had volunteered to take part. Some of them had previous experience of psychological interventions. However, this does suggest that experienced, specialist nurses who are motivated to develop and improve their skills do have the potential to deliver specific psychological therapies. It is also important to note that in addition to training, the nurses were given ongoing specialist supervision.

Outcomes of studies of nurses using CBT techniques

There are also studies that measure the outcome of nursing interventions using CBT-based techniques. A randomized controlled trial (RCT) was carried out to establish the advantages of Problem Solving Therapy (PST) given by community nurses compared to usual care by the GP. Seventy adult patients with anxiety, tension, depression, irritability, sleep disturbance or unexplained somatic symptoms of a minimum of four weeks duration were assigned to a PST or control group. Six community nurses were trained in PST. This included four half-day workshops, plus a period of practice supervision. The training was effective in developing competence but only after the supervised practice with patients. In terms of clinical outcomes, there was no difference between the groups, as assessed by various mood assessment instruments. However, the treated group showed less sickness days off work (Mynors-Wallis et al 1997).

In a pilot study within a cancer treatment centre, a novel multicomponent intervention by a nurse was evaluated. All patients were screened for a major depressive disorder, and cases of depression were allocated to either treatment as usual ($n = 31$) or to the intervention nurse ($n = 64$). The nurse, who had a background in cancer nursing, received six months training, was rated as competent and thereafter had weekly supervision. Up to ten sessions were given to each patient in the intervention group. This included education about depression and PST. Some of the patients in each group also had antidepressants prescribed by their GP. There were statistically significant improvements in depression scores at three and six months in the treated group (Sharpe et al 2004).

This study was further developed in a randomized trial at the same cancer centre. Two hundred patients with cancer who met criteria for a major depressive disorder were involved. One hundred and one were allocated to usual treatment, and 99 to the intervention group. The intervention involved up to 10 sessions of manualized PST, and education about depression and its treatment, given by three specially trained cancer nurses. Some patients in both groups were also given antidepressants by their GPs, but those in the intervention group were more likely to receive a therapeutic dose. The reduction in depressive symptoms was greater in the intervention group at six and twelve months, and there was also a greater reduction in anxiety and fatigue in this group at three months (Strong et al 2008).

Within a specialist palliative care context there is also evidence for the effectiveness of CBT. Moorey et al (2009) evaluated the effects of CBT training on the development of nurses' knowledge, and its impact on patients' symptoms. Fifteen home care clinical nurse specialists attended a two-day introductory workshop, followed by seven one-day workshops. They then had weekly supervision for a period of one year before the start of the trial. Their skills were assessed at the end of the training year and three months after randomization for the trial. Competence was rated higher in the intervention group (statistically significant for 7 of 10 items) than in a control group of nurses. In terms of interventions, a sample of 80 patients were allocated to the CBT group ($n = 45$) or treatment as usual ($n = 35$). Within the intervention group, anxiety scores were lower, but depression scores were the same as the control group at 16 weeks.

Overall, these studies give a clear picture of the potential for adult general nurses, if motivated and given specialist education, to deliver psychological interventions that are targeted at their patient group. This is true of PST, and more general training in CBT techniques is also effective. There is also some emerging evidence of the effectiveness of training in motivational interviewing.

Reflection point

- Within your own area of nursing practice, is there any evidence of the potential for nurses to deliver psychotherapeutic interventions?
- Is this an area of practice that you would be interested in developing?
- What skills and training do you think you would need to be able to practise in this area?
- What conditions would be necessary within your place of work to enable this to happen?

Summary

This chapter has discussed the potential for nurses to develop their work using psychotherapeutic models and techniques. The following chapters explore the most common psychosocial problems encountered in nursing practice, with discussions of their nature, assessment, management and nursing care, including the potential for nurses to develop their role further.

Key points

- There are limits to the practice of counselling in nursing but nurses can use counselling skills effectively in their practice;
- Psychodynamic psychotherapy is a complex and difficult therapy for nurses to practise but has many useful concepts that can be used in nursing;
- CBT is an effective and accessible form of psychotherapy that can be applied by nurses after training and with supervision;
- PST and motivational interviewing have proven potential for use by nurses, particularly in specialist care settings.

References

Baer, R. (2003) Mindfulness training as a clinical intervention: a conceptual and empirical review, *American Psychological Association*, 10 (2), 125–143.

Barnes, E., Griffiths, P., Ord, J. and Wells, D. (1998) *Face to Face with Distress. The Professional Use of Self in Psychosocial Care.* Oxford: Butterworth-Heinemann.

Beck, A., Rush, A., Shaw, B. and Emery, G. (1979) *Cognitive Therapy of Depression.* New York: Guilford Press.

Bottorff, J. and Morse, J. (1994) Identifying types of attending: patterns of nurses' work, *IMAGE: Journal of Nursing Scholarship*, 26 (1), 53–60.

Britt, E., Hudson, S. and Blampied N. (2004) Motivational interviewing in health settings: a review, *Patient Education and Counselling*, 53, 147–155.

Casement, P. (1985) *On Learning from the Patient.* Hove: Brunner-Routledge.

Cort, E., Moorey, S., Hotopf, M., Kapari, M., Monroe, B. and Hansford, P. (2009) Palliative care nurses' experiences of training in cognitive behaviour therapy and taking part in a randomised controlled trial, *International Journal of Palliative Nursing*, 15 (6), 290–298.

de Raeve, L., Rafferty, M. and Paget, M. (2009) *Nurses and their Patients: Informing Practice through Psychodynamic insights.* Cumbria: M&K Publishing.

Dryden, W. and Feltham, C. (eds) (1992) *Psychotherapy and its Discontents.* Buckingham: Open University Press.

Greenberger, D. and Padesky, C.A. (1995) *Mind Over Mood.* New York: Guilford Press.

Holmes, J. (1993) *John Bowlby and Attachment Theory.* London: Routledge.

Jones, A. (2005) Transference, counter-transference and repetition: some implications for nursing practice, *Journal of Clinical Nursing*, 14, 1177–1184.

Kitson, A. (1993) Formalizing concepts relating to nursing and caring, in Kitson, A. (ed.) *Nursing: Art and Science.* London: Chapman & Hall, pp. 25–47.

Maissi, E., Ridge, K., Treasure, J., Chalder, T., Roche, S., Bartlett, J., Schmidt, U., Thomas, S. and Ismail, K. (2011) Nurse-led psychological interventions to improve diabetes control: assessing competencies, *Patient Education and Counselling,* 84, e37–e43.

Mannix, K.A. et al (2006) Effectiveness of brief training in cognitive behaviour therapy techniques for palliative care practitioners, *Palliative Medicine,* 20 (6); 579–584.

Miller, W.R. and Rollnick, S. (2002) *Motivational Interviewing: Preparing People for Change* (2nd edition). New York: Guilford Press.

Moorey, S., Greer, S., Bliss, J. and Law, M. (1998) A comparison of adjuvant psychological therapy and supportive counselling in patients with cancer, *Psycho-oncology,* 7, 218–228.

Moorey, S., Cort, E., Kapari, M., Monroe, B., Hansford, P., Mannix, K., Henderson, M., Fisher, L. and Hotopf, M. (2009) A cluster randomised controlled trial of cognitive behaviour therapy for common mental disorders in patients with advanced cancer, *Psychological Medicine,* 39, 713–723.

Morriss, R., Gask, L., Smith, C. and Battersby, L. (1999) Training practice nurses to assess and manage anxiety disorders: a pilot study, *NT Research,* 4 (2), 132–142.

Mynors-Wallis, L., Davies, I., Gray, A., Barbour, F. and Gath, D. (1997) A randomised controlled trial and cost analysis of problem-solving treatment for emotional disorders given by community nurses in primary care, *British Journal of Psychiatry,* 170, 113–119.

Ramos, M.C. (1992) The nurse–patient relationship: theme and variations, *Journal of Advanced Nursing,* 17, 496–506.

Rogers, C. (2004) *On Becoming a Person: a Therapist's View of Psychotherapy.* London: Coustelle.

Roth, A. and Fonagy, P. (2005) *What Works for Whom?* (2nd edition). London: Guilford Press.

Sharpe, M., Strong, V., Allen, K., Rush, R., Maguire, P., House, A., Ramirez, A. and Cull, A. (2004) Management of major depression in outpatients attending a cancer centre: a preliminary evaluation of a multicomponent cancer nurse-delivered intervention, *British Journal of Cancer,* 90, 310–313.

Strong, V., Sharpe, M., Cull, A., Maguire, P., House, A. and Ramirez, A. (2004) Can oncology nurses treat depression? A pilot project, *Journal of Advanced Nursing,* 46 (5), 542–548.

Strong, V., Waters, R., Hibberd, C., Murray, G., Wall, L., Walker, J., McHugh, G., Walker, A. and Sharpe, M. (2008) Management of depression for people with cancer (SMaRT oncology 1): a randomised trial, *The Lancet,* 372, 40–48.

Westbrook, D., Kennerley, H. and Kirk, J. (2007) *An Introduction to Cognitive Behaviour Therapy: Skills and Applications.* London: SAGE Publications.

Williams, M., Teasdale, J., Segal, Z. and Kabat-Zinn, J. (2007) *The Mindful Way Through Depression: Freeing Yourself from Chronic Unhappiness.* Oxford: Oxford University Press.

Further reading

Mynors-Wallis, L. (2005) *Problem-solving Treatment for Anxiety and Depression: A Practical Guide.* Oxford: Oxford University Press.

Rollnick, S., Miller, W. and Butler, C. (2008) *Motivational Interviewing in Health Care: Helping Patients Change Behavior.* London: Guilford Press.

6

WORKING WITH THE ANXIOUS PERSON

Learning objectives

By the end of this chapter, you should be able to:

- understand the nature of anxiety as a mental health problem and as a personal experience;
- recognize the features of anxiety and undertake a basic assessment;
- respond with calmness and sensitivity to the person who is anxious, demonstrating understanding of their condition in the planning and delivery of nursing care;
- provide straightforward anxiety management and refer on for specialist management when necessary.

Introduction

Anxiety is a very common and familiar human experience. It has an evolutionary role by increasing vigilance in the individual and thereby protecting against potential threats in the environment. However, anxiety can also be quite distressing and disabling if it becomes very intense or persistent. Dealing effectively with anxiety is called anxiety management and this is a straightforward approach that can be incorporated into nursing care.

Understanding the nature and experience of anxiety

Experiences of feelings like anxiety and fear are commonplace. The two emotions are related but there are differences. Fear relates to an actual threat and anxiety is a response to the possibility of threat. For example, if you start crossing a road at a pedestrian crossing and a fast car comes towards you, you are likely to feel fear. However, if you feel unable to step onto the crossing because of apprehension that a car may hit you, then that is anxiety.

When is anxiety 'normal' and when does it become a problem?

Anxiety is an everyday experience for most people, and many situations provoke a degree of anxiety. 'Normal' anxiety can be seen as a means of evoking a coping response to deal with a perception of threat. If there is a successful coping reaction, then the threat is resolved and the anxiety subsides (Westbrook et al 2011).

As long as we feel we are able to manage the problem triggering the anxiety, and we feel in control, anxiety does not have to be a problem. Anxiety becomes a problem when it is distressing, it feels out of control, or it stops us carrying on with our life as normal. This may be because of its severity. A panic attack is an acute episode of severe anxiety that can be quite disabling as well as frightening. Anxiety that has a long duration, for example more than a few hours, can be exhausting. Also, anxiety can be a problem because of its specific effects. For example, anxiety about going to hospital could lead to an important appointment being missed.

Different people have different levels of anxiety in their day-to-day lives. For some people, a high level or constant presence of anxiety is a normal part of life. This is sometimes referred to as 'trait' anxiety, as opposed to 'state' anxiety, that is, anxiety stimulated by factors in the environment. Worry is also part of many people's normal experience of life. Worry is a way in which they attempt to cope or problem-solve, by thinking about something in depth and over time. It can become a problem if it is associated with distress or negative feelings, it feels out of control or the worry itself becomes a source of anxiety, that is, worrying about worry (Wells 1997).

Reflection point

Think of a patient you have nursed who had a problem with anxiety. What was it about their circumstances that contributed to their anxiety? Did it have any impact on the way that you provided nursing care?

In essence, anxiety is not a problem if it is effective in maintaining the individual's ability to cope. If it is excessive or inappropriate and it fails to aid the resolution of problems, it can become a problem itself, and often this becomes established as a cyclical pattern for people whose coping is ineffective. This is illustrated in Figure 6.1.

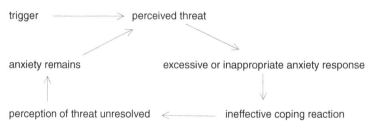

Figure 6.1 Modelling anxiety: cognitive model of problem anxiety
Source: adapted from Westbrook et al 2011

Panic attacks

Panic attacks are a specific form of anxiety where the anxiety is both severe and acute. It generally has the following features:

- hyperventilation, shortness of breath;
- strong physical sensations of anxiety; for example, palpitations, chest pain;
- fearful, catastrophic thoughts of death, madness or losing control;
- a sense of impending doom.

In addition to hyperventilation and tachycardia, people can experience choking sensations, dizziness, numbness or tingling in the fingers and toes. These strong physical sensations and acute sense of dread often lead to fears that a catastrophic health event is taking place, for example myocardial infarction or cerebrovascular accident. This can lead to a selective focus on the physical sensations, which then perpetuates the panic attack. Isolated panic attacks, where the trigger event can be identified, are relatively straightforward to manage. However, panic disorder, where attacks become frequent and there is no single identifiable cause, can be more complex and difficult to treat.

Health anxiety

Health anxiety is a form of anxiety disorder where the focus of the anxiety is the person's health. In its milder forms, it can take the form of a preoccupation with health and a tendency to *misinterpret common symptoms* as something more serious for example a headache as a sign of a brain tumour. In more serious cases, also called *hypochondriasis*, there is an ongoing obsession with the possibility of serious illness, in spite of evidence to the contrary. This can involve persistent checking for and reporting of symptoms that cause concern to the individual as evidence of serious illness. There may be features of panic, obsessive thoughts, or depression.

Health anxiety is an important condition for nurses to be aware of, as it may lead to unnecessary investigations, inaccurate diagnoses and inappropriate treatments, in addition to considerable distress for the patient. Underlying health anxiety is an erroneous or mistaken health belief (e.g. chest pain means you are having a heart attack) and a tendency to interpret physical sensations as confirmation that these beliefs are realistic (see Figure 6.2).

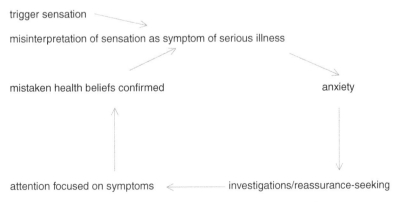

Figure 6.2 Modelling anxiety: cognitive model of health anxiety
Source: adapted from Westbrook et al 2011

Anxiety, stress and trauma

Anxiety is a response to stress or uncertainty. Within the context of health care, there are countless stressful situations that can provoke anxiety, including the health problem itself, treatment and the health care environment (see Box 6.1). Severe stress can trigger stress or trauma conditions, which by their nature are more severe and can be disabling if they persist (see Box 6.2). These are characterized by the following:

- Re-experiencing of the event in some form, for example, images, memories, dreams.
- Avoidance of associations with the event, for example, places, people.
- Increased arousal: anxiety, anger, sleep disturbance, hypervigilance.
- Significant distress or disability.

Sometimes people also experience the effects of stress as *detachment* and *numbness*, *depersonalization* (loss of the sense of being a separate individual, like watching oneself from the outside) or *derealization* (a sense that the external world does not seem real). *Acute stress reactions and disorders* may resolve without specific interventions. However, it is important for nurses to know about them in order that they can be supportive and understand the nature of the patient's experience.

Some acute stress disorders will progress to *post-traumatic stress disorder* (PTSD), so it is also very important that nurses recognize its features and are aware of how to refer on for specialist help. PTSD is increasingly being recognized as a consequence of common health care events, including childbirth (Lapp et al 2010), accidents, including traffic accidents (Kuch et al 1996), periods of time in the intensive care unit (Davydow et al 2008) and other medical conditions including heart disease (Tedstone and Tarrier 2003).

PTSD is also associated with military personnel who have experienced combat situations, health care personnel who attend accidents or other professionals who deal with violent or stressful events, such as the police. A history of rape, sexual assault or childhood abuse can also lead to the development of PTSD. Untreated, PTSD can be very long-lasting and disabling, and can be associated with alcohol and drug misuse, and other long-term health problems, including anxiety and depression. It is treatable, and cognitive behavioural therapy (CBT) is particularly effective.

Box 6.1 Examples of stressful events and situations in health care

Acute health care settings
- Traumatic events that lead to hospital admission (e.g. accidents)
- Waiting in A&E
- Time in intensive care (critical care)

Surgery
- The anaesthetic
- Pain and discomfort
- The operation
- Being unconscious

(Mitchell 2005)

Long-term conditions
- Being given bad news
- Investigations and waiting for test results
- Changes in body image
- Uncertainty

Box 6.2 Stress and trauma conditions

Acute stress reaction is short term, lasting only a few hours or days

Acute stress disorder lasts from two days to four weeks

- Both acute stress reaction and disorder can present with distress, agitation, anxiety, numbing, detachment, derealization or depersonalization

Post-traumatic stress disorder (PTSD) if symptoms persist beyond one month

- Flashbacks, anger, anxiety, long-term health problems.

Links with other physical health problems

Pain

Anxiety increases sensitivity to pain and body sensations. Anxiety will therefore make the experience of pain more intense and more difficult to manage. The *meaning* attached to the pain is a very significant factor in determining how the individual will cope with the pain. A contributory factor to problems coping with pain is *catastrophizing*, a tendency to expect the worst possible outcome. This may turn the experience of pain from *uncomfortable* to *unbearable*.

Depression

Anxiety is often present in people who are depressed, and depression can present with features of anxiety or agitation, particularly more severe cases. Anxiety commonly occurs with both fatigue and depression.

Breathlessness

There is a very close link between breathlessness and anxiety, and there is a physiological basis for this. Hypoxia can trigger anxiety and anxiety is associated with the rapid, shallow breathing (hyperventilation) that is a feature of panic attacks. Breathlessness can be effectively treated with a combination of support, education and anxiety management (Bredin et al 1999). It is always important to identify any physical cause for breathlessness before managing the anxiety associated with it.

Long-term conditions

Long-term conditions, by their nature, involve stressful events and longer-term stressful situations, variations in health status and difficult symptom experiences. This involves a degree of illness uncertainty, the need to deal with and make sense of an uncertain future (Mast 1998).

Cancer

Anxiety about cancer recurrence, 'check-up anxiety', is a common feature of the experience of cancer, and is identified as a fundamental aspect of cancer survivorship (Doyle 2008). This can lead to a state of *hypervigilance*, where the patient is constantly alert to the possibility of recurrence, and may interpret any ache, pain or lump as a sign that this is happening. In the case of cancer, there is the additional burden of its association in the public awareness with death and suffering. While this is not always a realistic appraisal of the nature of the condition, it will inevitably have an impact on the mind of the person with cancer, facing them with their own mortality and the possibility of their own death. Disproportionate fear of death may be termed *death anxiety*, and this is probably one end of a continuum of the existential anxieties that we all face.

Types of anxiety diagnosis

Panic disorder

This is characterized by recurrent acute attacks of severe anxiety. These are not associated with any specific trigger event or situation. Physically, the individual can experience hyperventilation and palpitations, chest pain and feelings of depersonalization or derealization. Psychologically, the person experiences intense feelings of fear or dread, and may fear that they are dying or going mad.

Generalized anxiety disorder

This is a form of generalized worry, sometimes referred to as *free-floating anxiety* as it is not attached to or triggered by specific circumstances. The individual can experience a range of anxiety symptoms; for example, nervousness, tension, palpitations, dizziness and physical discomfort. It may be associated with a fear that something bad is going to happen.

Phobic anxiety disorders or phobias

This includes a range of disorders where the anxiety is precipitated by very specific triggers. This can lead to avoidance of these triggers or very strong feelings of anxiety when they are encountered. An example is *social phobia* or *social anxiety*, a fear of the disapproval of others that can be linked to feelings of low self-esteem or fear of criticism (in some cases linked to altered body image). *Needle phobia* is a form of anxiety that can make it difficult for people to accept treatment or attend hospitals.

Obsessive compulsive disorder (OCD)

OCD is associated with recurrent obsessional thoughts or compulsions. Obsessional thoughts are distressing thoughts, images or impulses that keep entering the individual's mind in spite of attempts to resist them. Compulsions are acts or rituals that are performed out of a feeling that they prevent something bad happening. The individual is aware that these actions are pointless but cannot resist the compulsion without experiencing anxiety.

Assessment

The assessment of anxiety is based on physical, psychological and behavioural factors.

Physical assessment

The presentation of anxiety can be very visual: flushing, perspiration and agitation are common. Although we think of anxiety as a psychological condition, anxiety has very many physical features (see Box 6.3), associated with arousal of the autonomic nervous system. An important aspect of the assessment of anxiety is recognizing these and eliminating a treatable physical cause (see Box 6.4). This is also an important aspect of nursing care: educating the patient to recognize the physical features of anxiety, which can be misinterpreted and attributed to physical illness; for example, tachycardia may be interpreted as a sign of heart disease. This is more likely in people prone to health anxiety, or people with a pre-existing health condition, who may be vigilant and looking for signs of worsening of their disease. However, other causes of tachycardia and hyperventilation should always be considered in assessment.

Box 6.3 Physical features of anxiety

- Tachycardia
- Hyperventilation
- Muscular tension
- Fatigue
- Pains (e.g. head, stomach)
- Perspiration
- Flushing
- Pallor
- Tremor
- Nausea
- Diarrhoea
- Frequency of urination

Box 6.4 Physical causes of anxiety

Organic
- Respiratory disorders (e.g. COPD)
- Metabolic conditions (e.g. hypoxia)
- Neurological conditions (e.g. delirium)
- Endocrine disorders (e.g. hypoglycaemia)
- Cardiovascular disorders (e.g CCF)

Drugs
- Corticosteroids, bronchodilators
- Drug and alcohol withdrawal

Psychological assessment

The central psychological feature of anxiety is a sense of apprehension or dread (see Box 6.5). Anxiety can make it more difficult to concentrate, perform tasks and to make decisions. The individual may feel tense, nervous or 'on edge'. Thoughts may be scary or obsessive, characterized by worry and ruminating, that is, recurrent thinking about topics. Another feature of anxiety can be selective attention, focusing on the specific stimuli that are a cause for concern.

Behavioural assessment

People who are anxious may be tense, agitated or restless. Their behaviour may be different from normal, in that tension and irritability may make them sensitive and edgy or fear and vulnerability may lead to reassurance-seeking behaviour (see Box 6.6).

Box 6.5 Psychological features of anxiety

- Poor concentration
- Difficulty making decisions
- Worrying thoughts
- Irritability
- Fearfulness, apprehension, uncertainty
- A sense of impending doom
- Fears of loss of control, serious illness, death, going mad

---

Box 6.6 Behavioural features of anxiety

- Agitation
- Restlessness, pacing
- Seeking reassurance
- Avoidance of anxiety-provoking situations
- Sleep and appetite disturbance

Assessment tools

Assessment tools are a useful way of screening for anxiety. A suspicion of a clinical level of anxiety after using assessment and screening tools should lead to a referral to a qualified mental health specialist.

Distress thermometer (Roth et al 1998)

The distress thermometer is a simple single item visual analogue scale that asks the question *'how distressed have you been during the past week on a scale of 0 to 10?'* This can be useful in assessing people whose ability to concentrate or cooperate with treatment is severely impaired.

Hospital Anxiety and Depression Scale (HADS) (Zigmond and Snaith 1983)

The HADS was developed for the purpose of assessing anxiety and depression in the physically ill. There are seven questions relating to anxiety, each with a potential score of 0–3. The anxiety scale is therefore 0–21. For screening purposes, clinical anxiety is considered to be present with a score of 11 and above. The HADS has the advantage of being quick and straightforward to fill in and to score.

Health Anxiety Inventory (HAI) (Salkovskis et al 2002)

This is a specialized questionnaire that can be used for detecting health anxiety in medical settings. The HAI is a 14-point questionnaire (there are also longer versions), with four potential statements in response to each question.

For a detailed discussion of anxiety assessment instruments, see Wells (1997).

Anxiety management

Nursing care of the anxious person

There are a number of actions the nurse can take to incorporate the principles of anxiety management into nursing care (see Box 6.7).

Helping the patient feel in control

If anxiety is a response to uncertainty or feeling out of control, then supporting the patient to feel more in control is the logical intervention, and there is theoretical and empirical support for this. Both external factors, including the nature of the support offered, and internal factors, such as feelings of optimism, self-efficacy and an internal locus of control (a sense that control is located within, rather than outside, of the person) have a significant effect on whether anxiety will be reduced (Mitchell 2005). All activities that enhance the feeling of control of the patient, and their family, will enhance anxiety management. This includes offering choices at all stages of care and treatment, involvement in decision-making, identifying concerns and responding to the patient's priorities.

Providing reassurance by acting confidently and containing the anxiety

Reassurance has the potential to instil confidence by providing the optimal conditions for care, enhancing patient control and reducing uncertainty (Teasdale 1995). Acts that promote confidence and comfort, for example, a reassuring touch on the arm, rearranging bedding, getting a drink, are a first step towards instilling confidence. Confidence is built by actions that are professional in manner, demonstrate understanding of the patient's condition, and actions to relieve discomfort and distress. Working with anxious people can be difficult if the nurse finds it difficult to be calm and effective in the face of stress or distress. *Containment* is a term from psychodynamic psychotherapy (see Chapter 5) that gives us a model for understanding how anxiety or distress can be 'held' by the nurse. This means that the nurse needs to model a calm, confident approach to the cause of the anxiety and to its resolution.

Acting effectively to deal with treatable causes of anxiety

Treatable causes include both physical factors that are reversible (see Box 6.4 – Physical causes of anxiety), and anxiety where there is a clear psychosocial cause, for example panic attacks associated with specific triggers. Effective treatment includes anxiety and panic first aid.

Demonstrating a professional understanding of anxiety and its management

Effective nursing care involves responding to the concerns that the patient and family have, and also responding to the effects of the anxiety. This involves demonstrating an understanding of what anxiety is and what its effects are, and the strategies that can be used to deal with it: anxiety management.

*Providing information in a manner, format and time that
is acceptable to the patient*

Not all patients want the same amount or type of information. It is therefore very important that information is available in different formats, and that people have some choice in the amount and the level of information that is offered. For example, verbal information can be supplemented by written information that will be available later when people have more time. An initial offer of information can be reviewed to see how this has been received and what remaining questions the individual has. Information-giving is not a single event. People need time, particularly if they are anxious, to take in, process and retain information.

Health education

Anxiety is an aspect of health, and an understanding of its nature and effects should be incorporated into health education. As the underlying function of (healthy) anxiety is to promote coping, then education about coping strategies and anxiety management is an effective form of health education.

Reflection point

Can you recall an experience of caring for a person who was anxious? Do you recall aspects of their care that were effective, and those that were not effective? On reflection, would you plan their care differently now?

Box 6.7 Key features of nursing care of the anxious person

- Helping the patient feel in control
- Providing reassurance by acting confidently and containing the anxiety
- Acting effectively to deal with treatable causes of anxiety
- Demonstrating a professional understanding of anxiety and its management
- Providing information in a manner, format and time that is acceptable to the patient
- Health education

Anxiety and panic first aid

This section describes how to manage acute anxiety, particularly when associated with panic and hyperventilation. There are two elements to this: the management of the physical symptoms, particularly breathing, and cognitive management.

Managing breathing

Hyperventilation is a vicious cycle of overbreathing, reduced blood carbon dioxide through expiration, and a resulting sense of breathlessness and dizziness that accentuates the anxiety. People who are overbreathing may not realize what is causing the problem; they are too focused on their worrying thoughts. First, explain to the patient what is happening, that the overbreathing is keeping the anxiety going and that the breathing needs to be brought under control. Ask the patient to breathe in through their nose. This has the effect of making breathing more noticeable, and it slows it down. Ask the patient to focus on their breathing, and to slow it down and deepen it. It helps to ask them to place a hand on the chest, and on the stomach, above the diaphragm. They can then watch the rise and fall of the ribs and diaphragm, making breathing a visible process. You can also model this yourself, breathing slowly and deeply, asking the patient to keep up a similar pace. This intervention includes all of the key elements of nursing care of the anxious patient: providing reassurance and containment, showing understanding and dealing with the causes of anxiety, enabling patient control, providing information and health education (see Box 6.8).

Box 6.8 Managing breathing

- Explain what is happening
- Breathe through the nose
- Focus on the breathing
- Breathe slowly and deeply
- Hand on chest and stomach

Cognitive management of acute anxiety

If the physical aspects of acute anxiety have been effectively managed, you can move on to deal with the cognitive elements. In order to do this it is helpful to understand the cognitive model of panic. This involves a trigger event, which may be a sensation (e.g. shortness of breath), an image (e.g. seeing someone who is very ill), emotion (e.g. fear) or a situation (e.g. being in hospital). This precipitates an anxious thought or thoughts, for example, 'I am going to die', leading to anxiety and its associated symptoms. The anxiety is then worsened by the symptoms of anxiety, and hyperventilation will then lead to further symptoms. These symptoms can be misinterpreted as signs that something catastrophic is going to happen or that death is imminent. This is summarized below:

- trigger (sensation, image, emotion, situation);
- anxious thought(s);
- anxiety;
- body symptoms;

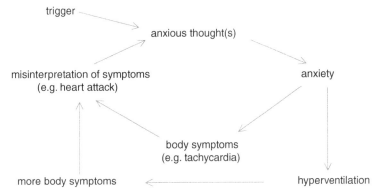

Figure 6.3 Modelling anxiety: cognitive model of panic

Source: adapted from *Understanding Panic* by David Westbrook and Khadija Rouf, published by Oxford Cognitive Therapy Centre (www.octc.co.uk)

- misinterpretation of symptoms;
- catastrophic interpretation of the situation.

Figure 6.3 illustrates this process.

Management therefore involves discussing with the patient what happened, and identifying triggers and anxious thoughts. The following questions are a guide to assessment:

- Can you describe the situation before the panic attack? Can you think yourself back into that situation?
- Where were you? What were you doing? Who were you with? What happened? Do you remember how you were feeling?
- What was going through your mind just before you began to panic? Do you remember any specific thoughts?
- What physical feelings and sensations did you have during the panic attack?

If it is possible to identify specific triggers and anxious thoughts, it will also be possible to prepare for these arising again. This gives the patient scope for control, and the patient can begin to understand the process of panic, reducing the potential for misinterpretation of feelings or sensations during any future panic attacks. The patient can also begin to develop preventive strategies for managing anxiety.

Anxiety management strategies

It is important for people to have a range of preventive strategies for managing anxiety. This is particularly helpful for people who regularly have problems with anxiety, but anyone who faces stressful and anxiety-provoking situations would benefit.

Relaxation

Being able to relax and to invoke a sense of relaxation in the face of stress is a powerful tool in the management of anxiety. Some people are more able to relax than others, but relaxation is a skill that can be learned. Some environmental factors promote a sense of well-being and relaxation, including physical comfort; for example, comfortable clothes, position and seating, a suitable room temperature and a lack of noise or disturbance. Music can be very relaxing, and this can be used to reduce anxiety during hospital procedures (Mitchell 2005).

Progressive muscle relaxation (PMR) is a way of tensing and relaxing groups of muscles in a progressive pattern (e.g. facial, neck, shoulders), focusing on the sensation produced by this. In this way, the individual learns to recognize the sense of relaxation, and develops the capacity to induce relaxation, for example by using a specific cue. *Cued relaxation* is triggered by a word, an object or symbol, and these can be chosen to represent an internal image or feeling of calm. For example, the word 'calm', the colour blue, or a pebble from a beach may represent calm and relaxation for an individual. This can also be combined with guided imagery, developing an internal mental image (e.g. a beach, the sky) that represents calm and positive energy.

Distraction is a way of refocusing the mind on an alternative to negative or worrying thoughts. This is different from avoidance, which is characterized by behaviours that prevent anxiety arising but fail to resolve it. Distraction techniques include:

- *external focus* – concentrating attention on the outside world, rather than internal preoccupations. Encourage patients to look at and notice, or describe, what they see around them, focusing particularly on pleasant and positive images.
- *physical exercise* – this needs to reflect the functional ability, fitness and energy of the patient, so this could include aerobic exercise, gentle stretching, or any household activity that provides distraction from worry.
- *mental exercises* – this can be similar to guided imagery in that the patient can distract themselves by a positive internal image. Alternatively, simply counting or repeating words from a poem or a song can help.

Case study: anxiety

Andrew Brown is a 45-year-old man who suffers from chronic obstructive pulmonary disease (COPD). The condition has limited his activity and he has not worked for several years. Recently, he has experienced quite severe episodes of breathlessness and anxiety. During these episodes, he becomes acutely breathless, hyperventilates, feels helpless and out of control, and experiences intense anxiety and dread. Andrew discusses these episodes with the practice nurse at his local health centre. He says he is afraid that his disease is out of control, and thinks it likely he will die during one of the episodes. His specialist nurse is familiar with his medical condition, and also knows about the links between panic attacks and breathlessness. She discusses the last episode in detail with him, while it is fresh in his mind, asking questions about how he felt just prior to and during the attack. He says he was gardening, and started to become breathless. The memory of the last episode crossed his mind as he felt a sudden rise in his level of anxiety. He started hyperventilating, and two thoughts rapidly crossed his mind: *I can't breathe* and *I'm going to die*. He felt an intense sense of dread as though something awful was about to happen. The nurse recognizes the symptoms of a panic attack and discusses this with Andrew, identifying differences from other causes of acute breathlessness. She talks him through managing his breathing, taking slow, deep breaths, and being more aware of the rise and fall of his chest and diaphragm. She then discusses how he can recognize anxious thoughts and distract himself by focusing on external images. Two weeks later he reports having had a panic attack and he tried the breathing and distraction exercises. This helped, and he has not had an episode of panic since.

Longer-term management strategies

In the longer term, people with anxiety problems can improve their ability to manage their anxiety by having psychotherapy, like CBT, and by developing their problem-solving capabilities and self-awareness. They can also manage their life in a more proactive way, managing personal time and resources, and developing personal assertiveness. There are many self-help books and other resources that can be recommended to patients to manage their lives in an effective way (see 'Self-help resources' below).

Treatment for anxiety disorders

In severe cases of anxiety, for example generalized anxiety disorder and obsessive compulsive disorder, anxiolytic medication such as benzodiazepines, or antidepressants including selective serotonin reuptake inhibitors (SSRIs) or serotonin norepinephrine reuptake inhibitors (SNRIs) can be an effective treatment. However, there is a limited role for medication in the management of anxiety in less severe cases. Anxiolytics have the capacity to develop dependency, and there may be other side effects from medication. They should therefore only be used in acute situations to manage anxiety in the short term. CBT is an effective treatment for a range of anxiety disorders.

Self-help resources

Books

Butler, G. and Hope, T. (2007) *Manage your Mind: The Mental Fitness Guide*. Oxford: Oxford University Press.

Kennerley, H. (2009) *Overcoming Anxiety*. London: Robinson.

Powell, T. (2000) *The Mental Health Handbook* (3rd edition). Milton Keynes: Speechmark Publishing Ltd.

Internet

Mind: www.mind.org.uk/help/medical_and_alternative_care/how_to_stop_worrying?

NHS Choices: www.nhs.uk/Conditions/Anxiety/Pages/self-help.aspx

University of Cambridge Counselling Service: www.counselling.cam.ac.uk/selfhelp/leaflets/anxiety

Summary

Although a universal phenomenon, anxiety can also be a severe and disabling condition. It is important to recognize when it is a problem for patients and to be able to undertake a screening assessment. Anxiety management techniques are accessible to both nurses and patients themselves. The next chapter deals with the other common psychological problem encountered in practice: depression.

Key points

- Anxiety is a common human experience in response to stress and uncertainty;
- It is associated with many health conditions and health care situations;
- Anxiety can become a problem if it becomes severe, long-lasting or causes distress;
- Symptoms of anxiety may be confused with other health problems, so recognition in practice and patient education are important;
- Some anxiety management techniques can be applied by nurses or patients themselves;
- Effective nursing care of people experiencing anxiety aids coping.

References

Bredin, M., Corner, J., Krishnasamy, M., Plant, H., Bailey, C. and A'Hern, R. (1999) Multi-centre randomised controlled trial of nursing intervention for breathlessness in patients with lung cancer, *British Medical Journal*, 318, 901.

Davydow, D., Gifford, J., Desai, S., Needham, D. and Bienvenu, J. (2008) Posttraumatic stress disorder in general intensive care unit survivors: a systematic review, *General Hospital Psychiatry*, 30, 421–434.

Doyle, N. (2008) Cancer survivorship: evolutionary concept analysis, *Journal of Advanced Nursing*, 62, 499–509.

Kuch, K., Cox., B. and Evans, R. (1996) Posttraumatic stress disorder and motor vehicle accidents: a multidisciplinary overview, *Canadian Journal of Psychiatry*, 41 (7): 429–434.

Lapp, L., Agbokou, C., Peretti, C. and Ferreri, F. (2010) Management of post traumatic stress disorder after childbirth: a review, *Journal of Psychosomatic Obstetrics & Gynaecology*, 31 (3), 113–122.

Mast, M.E. (1998) Survivors of breast cancer: illness uncertainty, positive reappraisal, and emotional distress, *Oncology Nursing Forum*, 25 (3), 555–562.

Mitchell, M. (2005) *Anxiety Management in Adult Day Surgery: A Nursing Perspective*. London: Whurr.

Roth, A., Kornblith, A., Batel-Copel, L. et al (1998) Rapid screening for psychologic distress in men with prostate carcinoma: a pilot study, *Cancer*, 82, 1904–1908.

Salkovskis, P., Rimes, K., Warwick, H. and Clark, D. (2002) The Health Anxiety Inventory: development and validation of scales for the measurement of health anxiety and hypochondriasis, *Psychological Medicine*, 32, 843–853.

Teasdale, K. (1995) Theoretical and practical considerations on the use of reassurance in the nursing management of anxious patients, *Journal of Advanced Nursing*, 22 (1), 79–86.

Tedstone, J. and Tarrier, N. (2003) Posttraumatic stress disorder following medical illness and treatment, *Clinical Psychology Review*, 23, 409–448.

Wells, A. (1997) *Cognitive Therapy of Anxiety Disorders: A Practice Manual and Conceptual Guide*. Chichester: John Wiley & Sons.

Westbrook, D. and Rouf, K. (1998) *Understanding Panic* (2nd edition). Oxford: Oxford Cognitive Therapy Centre.

Westbrook, D., Kennerley, H. and Kirk, J. (2011) *An Introduction to Cognitive Behaviour Therapy: Skills and Applications* (2nd edition). London: Sage Publications.

Zigmond, A.S. and Snaith, R.P. (1983) The Hospital Anxiety and Depression Scale, *Acta Psychiatrica Scandinavica*, 67, 361–370.

7

WORKING WITH THE DEPRESSED PERSON

Learning objectives

By the end of this chapter, you should be able to:

- understand the nature of depression as a mental health condition and as a personal experience;
- recognize the features of depression and undertake a basic assessment;
- respond with respect and sensitivity to the person who is depressed, demonstrating understanding of their condition in the planning and delivery of nursing care;
- know how depression is treated and how to refer on for specialist management where necessary.

Introduction and learning objectives

Depression is a very common and debilitating condition. Fifteen per cent of all people will have a depressive episode during their lifetime, the rate being higher in women. In primary care, 5–10 per cent of all patients have a major depression, and in the physically ill, particularly those with long-term conditions, rates of depression increase to 20 per cent and above. There is considerable overlap with other health conditions such as anxiety and pain. Depression can be very distressing, to the person who experiences it and to those around them. Depression has a profound impact on quality of life. Depression alone leads to a worse quality of life than most long-term conditions, and where the two are found together, it is even worse (Moussavi et al 2005). In the context of nursing care, it is a condition that can be recognized and helped.

Understanding the nature and experience of depression

Although depression is common, it is not a universal human experience. Unlike anxiety, not everyone becomes depressed, though most people will experience some features of depression, for example loss of interest and pleasure in things, sleep and appetite disturbance, at some time in their lives. A more universal and familiar human experience is sadness, and it is important to distinguish between depression and sadness to identify what may be a 'normal', transitory reaction to life events on the one hand, and what is a more serious, disabling and treatable condition on the other.

We can think of sadness as a short-term reaction to distressing life events. It is understandable and usually in proportion to the situation, though individuals will react differently depending on their interpretation of the nature of the event. Personality also has an impact: people who are sad may choose to bear it alone, or they may welcome the support of family and friends. When we are sad, our mood can lift in response to positive events, and we can enjoy life. Sadness does not need specialist help. In contrast, depression tends to be more severe and persistent, does not vary in response to events and may not spontaneously get better (see Table 7.1).

Reflection Point

Think of a patient you have nursed who was diagnosed with depression. What do you remember about their experience of the depression? What impact did it have on their life, and did it have an impact on their care?

In addition to these differences between sadness and depression, another way of understanding the difference is between levels of depression that are a cause for professional concern and intervention, and those that are not. Many people experience distressing features of depression, without reaching a level where depression can

Table 7.1 Differences between depression and sadness

Depression	Sadness
Feels outcast and alone	Able to feel intimately connected with others
The mood has a feeling of permanence	There is a feeling that some day this will end
Regretful, rumination on irredeemable mistakes	Able to enjoy happy memories
Extreme self-depreciation or self-loathing	Has a sense of self-worth
The mood is constant and unremitting	Sadness comes in waves
No hope, no interest in the future	Looks forward to things
Enjoys few activities	Retains capacity for pleasure
The presence of suicidal thoughts, suicidal behaviour	Has the will to live

Source: reprinted with permission from The Cicely Saunders Institute and the Institute of Psychiatry, King's College London: L. Rayner, A. Price, M. Hotopf, I.J. Higginson, The development of evidence-based European guidelines on the management of depression in palliative cancer care, 2011, 47, pp. 702–711.

be diagnosed. These can be termed *subthreshold depressive symptoms*. These may not warrant professional intervention, but can be managed by the individual using self-help literature or computerized material. More severe forms of depression, which can be diagnosed and treated by mental health professionals, are termed *major depression* or *clinical depression*.

As you can see from Table 7.1, depression is not just more severe than sadness, but there is a different quality to the experience of depression. It is an uncomfortable and unpleasant experience. People with depression experience a loss of the ability to experience emotion, and to experience a range of emotions, or *emotional blunting*. People with depression may describe feelings of numbness, being cut off from feelings, people and their surroundings. They may also describe their mood in terms of darkness, drowning or feeling trapped by their mood.

> I can remember particularly bad days. I would only take the day in ten minute chunks because that was it…Everything in my head was negative. And that I couldn't feel anything. I couldn't feel anything for my husband. I couldn't feel anything for the children. It was like being inside a very, very thick balloon and no matter how hard I pushed out, the momentum of the skin of the balloon would just push me back in.

> Interview 19 (available online at www.healthtalkonline.org/) © 2012 University of Oxford

A characteristic of depression is the negative patterns of thinking that people experience. This often involves interpreting events as having a negative meaning that they would not have if they were not depressed. These negative thoughts are important to recognize as they are amenable to treatment by cognitive behavioural therapy.

> And…your brain sort of leaps to conclusions about things and you think, well all my friends haven't phoned me, it's because they don't like me any more. Rather than my friends haven't phoned me because they're busy, or because their baby's sick, or they're busy at work or what have you.

> Interview 11 (available online at www.healthtalkonline.org/) © 2012 University of Oxford

Features of depression – physical, psychological and social

Depression has a number of features that can be used in the diagnosis of depression as a clinical condition. A number of these are physical features (see Box 7.1). Physical features of depression are important because they may be the first presentation of the problem in a health care setting, and it is easy to miss them. It is also important to take them into account during assessment, as the same features may also be present in physical illness. Physical features become more prominent as depression becomes more severe.

Box 7.1 Physical features of depression

- Feeling slowed up
- Problems sleeping
- Fatigue and lack of energy
- Changes to the menstrual cycle
- Loss of appetite and weight
- Constipation
- Aches and pains

Psychological features are the key characteristics of clinical depression. When assessing for depression in the physically ill, they are the most reliable elements of diagnosis. The central features of depression are persistent, unvarying low mood and loss of enjoyment of life (*anhedonia*). This and the other psychological features of depression are summarized in Box 7.2. Loss of interest, pleasure and enjoyment combined with a pessimistic outlook can make people feel that life is not worth living.

Box 7.2 Psychological features of depression (see also Box 7.6 on psychological assessment)

- Low mood
- Negative and pessimistic outlook on life
- Loss of interest and enjoyment
- Feelings of worthlessness and guilt
- Feeling helpless and hopeless

Depression is also a social condition in that it affects how people relate to others. The depressed person finds it difficult to experience and express emotions and this inhibits social relationships. In its milder forms, depression may make someone feel lonely and isolated, even in company. In more severe forms, the depressed person may misinterpret interpersonal communications, feel rejected and despised by others, and avoid people. Lack of social support is a factor in maintaining depression (see Box 7.3).

Box 7.3 Social features of depression

- Reduced social interaction
- Social withdrawal or avoidance of people

Degrees of depression

Depression is experienced at different levels or degrees (see Box 7.4). Mild depressive episodes may be characterized more by a deep sense of dissatisfaction, loss of motivation and an inability to enjoy or find purpose in life. People can carry on working and it may not be apparent they are depressed to anyone other than those closest to them. These episodes may be a reaction to a specific situation in the person's life, and may get better without professional help when circumstances improve (though not always).

Moderate depressive episodes often manifest with tension and irritability, so they are also more likely to impact on others and be associated with social withdrawal. The physical and psychological features of depression are also more likely to be present; for example, sleep and appetite disturbance, problems with concentration and feelings of worthlessness and hopelessness. It is likely that the ability to work will be affected.

Severe depression is very incapacitating, with a marked impact on the ability to maintain relationships and work. Physically, the person may be very slowed up or extremely anxious and agitated. They may neglect their personal appearance and hygiene. The face will often betray the underlying mood with a very drawn or fearful appearance. Appetite and sleep disturbance will lead to weight loss and exhaustion. Thoughts are often despairing and hopeless, and guilt and remorse may be dominant. Suicidal ideas are common. There may be psychotic features, like paranoid delusions.

Severely depressed people can see themselves as having a negative effect on those around them.

> ... I felt I was such a horrible person that I would contaminate anybody somehow by sitting, even sitting beside them, they would somehow be able to tell how awful I was if I sat beside them ... that sort of feeling of self-hatred and it was so painful. I had a feeling if they did talk to me, they'd only be doing it because they were sorry for me, I was absolutely convinced.

Interview 13 (available online at www.healthtalkonline.org/) © 2012 University of Oxford

---

Box 7.4 Degrees of depression

Mild depressive episode
- Loss of enjoyment, deep dissatisfaction and loss of purpose

Moderate depressive episode
- More depressive features and some severe
- Sleep disturbance and fatigue
- Tension and irritability, social withdrawal

Severe depressive episode
- Distressed and agitated, or markedly slowed up
- Depressive cognitions prominent
- Suicidal ideas, possibly active suicidal ideas
- Social and occupational functioning severely disrupted

Depression can also have positive effects

Although depression is a very unpleasant and disabling condition, some people feel that it can have positive effects on their lives in the longer term, if they are able to learn new ways of seeing the world and doing things.

> Recovery. I think it's not to get back to how you were before, because that was your old self and you want to be developing your new self, because life is about changes and if you try to hang onto all those old things, you are going to find it really, really difficult. You want to be learning new ways of thinking and doing things and that's what I see recovery as. I don't see it as a permanent thing, 'I've now recovered and I'll never have another bout of depression again'. It's like saying I'll never break my ankle again. I might break my ankle again.
>
> Louise (available online at www.healthtalkonline.org/) © 2012 University of Oxford

For many people, learning to see the world differently is a result of psychotherapy, for others it is all part of a journey of self-discovery.

Reflection point

Have you had personal experience, in yourself or someone else, of learning something positive from a difficult episode in life?

Links with other health conditions or problems

Anxiety

Many depressed people are also anxious, and some depressed states are associated with strong features of anxiety. This includes agitation in severe depression. There are also areas of overlap between anxiety and depression: poor concentration, fatigue, restlessness, tension and irritability, sleep and appetite disturbance can occur in both (see Chapter 6).

Sleep disturbance

Most people with depression experience disturbed sleep, and it is not always possible to determine which are the cause and the effect. There are three main patterns of sleep disturbance in depression:

* *Early morning wakening* This is where the person regularly wakes two hours or more earlier than normal, and cannot get back off to sleep. This is a key diagnostic feature of depression, and occurs in moderate to severe degrees of depression.

- *Early insomnia* This is when the person cannot get off to sleep. Often, they are troubled by worried thoughts. This is more characteristic of less severe forms of depression.
- *Hypersomnia* This is when the person sleeps more than usual.

Fatigue

There is a strong association between depression and fatigue. It is also a feature of other physical and psychological conditions, including anxiety, infections, neurological conditions, cancer, heart disease, sleep disorders and chronic fatigue syndrome. Fatigue is a complex and multifactorial problem. The main consideration in assessment of fatigue is the impact that it has on the life of the patient, noting any improvements resulting from adjustments in lifestyle, and it is important to identify any treatable causes.

Pain

Complaints of pain are very common in depression. Pain may be experienced as a feature of depression, or pains may be comorbid conditions. This can also be described as 'depression-pain syndrome'. Pain complaints in depression are associated with more intense and persistent pain and longer duration of pain. There are also likely to be more social, occupational and financial problems, and increased use of health care.

Loss: grief, bereavement

The experience of loss, in grief or bereavement, has some similarities with depression, but is generally thought to be a different experience. Grief is characterized by shock and numbness, anguish, sometimes anger, intense feelings of longing and preoccupation with thoughts of the deceased person. Sleep and appetite are often disturbed. Tearfulness and feelings of sadness are common. However, bereaved people can become depressed so it is important to be aware of features of depression in the bereaved. These are: feelings of guilt that are not related to the bereavement; problems functioning and getting on with life; marked social withdrawal; suicidal ideas; or severe hallucinations.

Childbirth

A brief, transient period of disturbed mood in the mother (and some fathers) is very common after childbirth. However, features of depression persisting for more than two weeks, with an onset within a month of the birth, are indicative of *postnatal* or *postpartum depression*. This may occur in 10–15 per cent of mothers. The features are not significantly different from other depressions, but are likely to include feelings of being overwhelmed or not feeling able to adequately care for the new baby. Following childbirth, women are also at risk of higher levels of anxiety and a small minority also experience a psychotic reaction.

Other conditions associated with depression

- Hypothyroidism
- Neurological conditions: Parkinson's disease, multiple sclerosis, brain malignancy
- All long-term conditions
- Cancer, particularly end stage.

Assessment

The diagnosis of depression is undertaken by mental health professionals. This is usually based on the criteria in the manuals *Diagnostic and Statistical Manual of Mental Disorders* (DSM-IV-TR), and *International Statistical Classification of Diseases and Related Health Problems* (ICD-10). For nurses who are not trained in mental health assessment, the primary role is in recognizing the features of depression, and undertaking an initial screening assessment to identify depression. The main challenge of assessment for depression in the physically ill is dealing with the overlap between features of physical disease and physical features of the depression.

Presentation

There are a number of ways that depression may be presented in a health care setting, where the first impression is that the problem is a physical one. For example, in primary care over half of patients with depression report physical symptoms only (Goldberg and Bridges 1988; see Box 7.5). The following are examples of presentations for which there should be suspicion of the presence of depression:

- chronic pain
- chronic fatigue
- sleep disturbance
- chronic constipation
- sexual dysfunction
- reduced appetite with weight loss
- multiple physical symptoms
- physical symptoms with marked distress
- health anxiety or morbid preoccupation with illness
- failure to respond to or comply with treatment
- signs of dementia with no organic changes (depressive pseudodementia)

It is important to suspect depression in any of the above presentations.

Box 7.5 Assessment for physical features of depression

- Reduced level of activity, being slowed up or agitated
- Reduced level of self-care
- Changes to appetite and weight
- Changes to bowel habit
- Sleep disturbance
- Depressed or fearful appearance

Psychological assessment

Psychologically, the most significant feature of depression is persistent, unvarying low mood. When working with people who have a physical illness, particularly if it is acute or a long-term condition, assessment should focus on those features of depression that are less likely to be caused by the physical condition itself (see Box 7.6). Psychological assessment under these circumstances should substitute usually reliable diagnostic physical features of depression with psychological features that are more reliable in the physically ill (Endicott 1984). So, disturbances of appetite, weight, fatigue and sleep are not reliable as they can be caused by physical illness. However, a fearful or depressed appearance, a lack of emotional reactivity, social withdrawal and depressive cognitions are reliable as they are not affected by the physical illness.

Box 7.6 Assessment for psychological features of depression

- Loss of motivation and spontaneity
- Lack of emotional reaction to events (emotional reactivity)
- Reduced interest, enjoyment of life and pleasure (*anhedonia*)
- Poor concentration and attention, reduced capacity for decision-making
- Persistent tearfulness (though crying is less common in more severe episodes)
- Loss of sexual interest
- Excessive guilt, remorse and pessimism (*depressive cognitions*)
- Suicidal ideas

Social assessment

The main social feature to look for in depression is social withdrawal or avoidance of people. This often leads to poor eye contact and problems establishing rapport. In the physically ill, care should be taken to allow for any effects of disability or loss of physical function. Involving the family and friends in the assessment process will help to identify changes to the social habits of the individual. They may also notice tension and irritable behaviour more readily than the depressed person. Feelings of being avoided, criticized or despised by others are also indicative of depression.

Assessment should, wherever possible, include assessment of the social support available to the patient. A lack of social support, and a lack of social resources, including finances, employment, adequate housing and transport, are all associated with a higher risk of depression, and are likely to maintain it and make it harder to treat. Any specific ongoing problems or recent trigger events should be identified.

Reflection point

What opportunities are there in your work environment for involving family and significant others in the process of assessment?

Assessment for suicide risk

Depression is a significant risk factor for suicide, so suicidal ideas should always be considered when making an assessment. Without experience in mental health assessment, nurses may lack confidence in asking questions about suicidal ideas and intention. People are often worried that talking about them will make suicide more likely. However, this is not the case. People who are considering suicide often feel very lonely and isolated, and sharing their feelings is more likely to decrease their sense of isolation. It is helpful to think of suicidal ideas as graded between passive and active, and to ask questions progressively. Asking questions about suicidal ideas should always be undertaken sensitively and with enough time.

Passive suicidal ideas

Passive suicidal ideas are when the person does not care whether they live or die, or would like to die but has no intention of acting on this. These ideas are relatively common in people with long-term conditions, or in very stressful situations, but they are usually transient. In isolation from other factors, they are not necessarily a cause for concern, but asking about them is a useful first step in suicide risk assessment. A suitable question to ask to assess for passive suicidal ideas is:

'Have you been feeling so bad that you do not want to go living?'

Active suicidal ideas

Active suicidal ideas or thoughts mean that the person would like to die and is considering this as a serious option. To assess for active suicidal ideas, you can ask:

'Have you thought about killing yourself?'

Active suicidal intention with planning

The risk of suicide becomes much more serious when the person has the clear intention to do something to end their life and has begun to make plans, or has actual plans in place to do this. These plans may include: making a will, making arrangements for after their death, making a choice of method of suicide, and a place and time. The following questions will help to identify these thoughts and plans:

'Do you intend to kill yourself?'
'Have you thought how you might do it?'
'Do you have plans to kill yourself?'

Suicidal ideas should always be taken seriously. The situation should be discussed urgently with other members of the team, and the person should be referred for specialist psychiatric help.

Reflection point

Do you have access to mental health personnel in your area of work? What options do you have for making a referral for mental health assessment?

Assessment tools

Most of the tools used for assessing depression are designed to be used for screening, that is, they are not considered to be diagnostic, but as an aid to assessment. A suspicion of depression as a result of any of the following assessment/screening tools should lead to a referral for specialist mental health assessment.

Single and double question assessment (Chochinov et al 1997)

There is some evidence that a single item screening question is as effective as more detailed screening tools. It is useful particularly where time is limited or the patient has limited physical and mental energy for participation in assessment.

'Are you depressed?'

The double item assessment enables more features of depression to be picked up. A positive answer to either question should lead to a referral for specialist assessment.

'During the last month, have you been bothered by feeling down, depressed or hopeless?'

'During the last month, have you been bothered by having little interest or pleasure in doing things?'

Distress thermometer (Roth et al 1998)

The distress thermometer is a simple single item visual analogue scale that asks the question *'how distressed have you been during the past week on a scale of 0 to 10?'* This can be useful in assessing people whose ability to concentrate or cooperate with treatment is severely impaired.

Hospital Anxiety and Depression Scale (HADS) (Zigmond and Snaith 1983)

The HADS was developed for the purpose of assessing anxiety and depression in the physically ill. It focuses on those features of depression that are independent of the impact of physical illness. There are seven questions relating to depression, each with a potential score of 0–3. The depression scale is therefore 0–21. For screening purposes, clinical depression is considered to be present with a score of 11 and above. The HADS has the advantage of being quick and straightforward to fill in and to score.

Edinburgh Postnatal Depression Scale (EPDS) (Cox et al 1987)

The EPDS was developed specifically for use with mothers during the postnatal period. There are 10 items each with a score of 0–3. Questions relate, for example, to loss of enjoyment, self-blame and thoughts of self-harm. Out of a potential score of 30, 10 or more indicates depression.

Patient Health Questionnaire (PHQ-9) (Kroenke et al 2001)

The Patient Health Questionnaire is a nine-item scale with each item scoring 0–3, with a potential maximum score of 27; 10–14 indicates moderate depression, and more than 14 suggests moderate to severe depression.

Reflection point

Are any of these assessment tools a practical choice for you to use in your area of work?

Management of depression

Nursing care of the depressed person

Engagement is very important in the care of the depressed patient. People, when depressed, become socially withdrawn, often feeling that they not a worthwhile person and that others should not waste their time on them. It is important therefore to demonstrate interest and show that they are worthwhile. Rapport can also be a problem to be overcome. The depressed person characteristically avoids eye contact and often looks down when you are talking to them. This should be managed sensitively, by showing concern and personal availability, offering opportunities to engage when the patient feels more comfortable with the situation.

It is important to show *empathy* for depressed people, with a focus on the person, and not the depressed mood. Cognitive therapy has shown us that people remain depressed when they become stuck in negative patterns of thinking about themselves, others and their future. Their attention is biased towards those events that confirm this negative view of the world. *Listening* to the patient can give them a sense of self-worth and provide opportunities for ventilating uncomfortable feelings. In turn, the nurse can offer a more positive outlook on the future, providing an alternative view that they may be able to see as their mood lifts. Empathetic care will take account of the patient's tiredness, lack of energy and motivation, and their sense of hopelessness and futility, while encouraging them to continue to do things.

Activity is an important factor both in preventing and in treating depression. There is evidence that physical activity has an antidepressant effect (Harvey et al 2010). Where there are limitations imposed on physical activity by illness, any purposeful and rewarding activity that can achieved will give the patient a sense of control over their life, and a sense of satisfaction and self-worth. Setting short-term, achievable goals is a very effective way of re-establishing a sense of personal agency and self-worth.

The *social context* of the patient may be an important factor in the development and maintenance of their condition. It is important to get to know and understand the patient's social circumstances, and mobilize any social support that they have access to.

It is essential to be aware of *the danger of suicide or self-harm* (see Chapter 9). Suicidal ideas should always be acted on by seeking specialist advice and consultation. Less urgent, but potentially critical in the longer term, is the danger of self-neglect. Maintaining personal hydration, diet, hygiene and appearance is a useful initial focus for activity in the depressed person. It may also be necessary to address the *sleep hygiene* of the patient (see Chapter 4).

Refer on for *mental health assessment* and treatment when necessary. Having done an initial screening assessment will give you confidence to make an effective referral to specialist services. Always discuss the referral with the patient (see Box 7.7).

Reflection point

Have you cared for a person who was clinically depressed? What went well, and what did not go well? On reflection, would you plan their care differently now?

Box 7.7 Key features of nursing care of the depressed person

- Engagement
- Empathy and listening
- Activity
- Awareness of the social context
- Awareness of self-harm and self-neglect
- Referral for specialist mental health assessment and treatment

Case study: depression

Carol Taylor is 55 years old and was diagnosed with breast cancer two years previously. She completed treatment some time ago, and has been informed that her illness has been successfully treated. Over the last two or three months, she has become low in mood, feeling uncomfortable with the effects of surgery and preoccupied with thoughts of the cancer coming back. She is sleeping poorly, waking more early than usual and feels tired all of the time. Her motivation and energy for work have reduced, and she is finding it hard to feel close to her family. Quite small things can provoke her to tears. At a follow-up appointment with the breast care nurse, she bursts into tears and tells her that she can't cope with life. The breast care nurse takes time to listen and shows empathy for Carol's situation. Recognizing the pattern of sleep disturbance, fatigue, loss of energy and motivation, emotional blunting and tearfulness, she suspects that Carol is depressed. She gives her the HADS to fill in and she scores 14 on the depression scale. The breast care nurse discusses this with Carol, who agrees that she feels depressed and would like some help. As the breast care nurse does not have direct access to specialist mental health services, she asks whether Carol would mind if she discussed a referral with her GP. Carol agrees this is a good idea, and says she will make an appointment to see her GP in the next week. The breast care nurse also discusses how things are at home, asking if she has been able to talk to her family or friends about how she is feeling.

Reflection point

Which other aspects of nursing care could the breast care nurse have addressed with Carol?

Psychotherapy for depression

The main form of psychotherapy for people with depression is cognitive behavioural therapy or cognitive therapy (CBT) (see Chapter 5). Some patients may also benefit from counselling or dynamic psychotherapy. The classic approach to CBT in depression is focused on activity scheduling and challenging negative assumptions (Beck et al 1979). *Activity scheduling* (recording and planning activity) gives opportunities to learn which activities give a sense of pleasure and a sense of achievement (for an example of activity recording see Figure 7.1, and also see Figure 7.2 for the cognitive model of depression on which this is based). Negative assumptions about the world, which contribute to the development and maintenance of depression, can be challenged by testing out in practice whether they are based in reality (behavioural experiments). However, CBT may need to be modified when working

Time/day	Monday	Tuesday	Wednesday	Thursday
8–9	Getting up, washed, breakfast (sad) P1 A3	Tired, in bed (sad) P1 A0	Get up, wash, no appetite (sad) P0 A3	Getting up, washed, breakfast (OK) P2 A5
9–10	Read papers (OK) P3 A2	Getting up, washed, breakfast (sad) P1 A3	Watch TV (sad) P1 A2	Clean living room (OK) P5 A
10–11	Washing up (feeling good) P5 A8	Watch TV (OK) P3 A2	Back to bed (hopeless) P1 A0	Friend visited (feeling good) P8 A5
11–12	Call Mum (OK) P6 A6	Shopping (OK) P3 A6	Bed (sad) P1 A0	Went out with friend for lunch (happy) P8 A8

Monitoring and recording daily activities and rating them for levels of pleasure and achievement:

- What I did (describe)
- How I felt (describe mood)
- Level of pleasure, P (0–10)
- Level of achievement, A (0–10)

Figure 7.1 Activity scheduling in depression

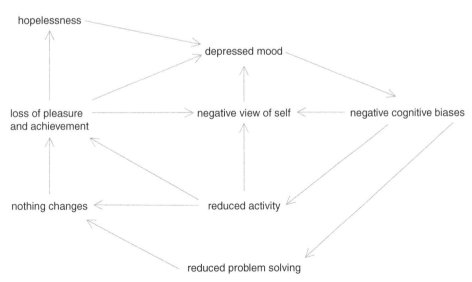

Figure 7.2 Cognitive model of depression

Source: adapted from Westbrook et al 2011

with people who have severe physical ill health, or whose condition is dynamic. For example, the potential for active planning may be hampered by changes in health status. CBT in people with a long-term condition like cancer will focus on the ventilation of feelings as well as dealing with underlying cognitive distortions (Moorey and Greer 2002).

Problem-solving is well established as a treatment for depression and there have been several studies of nurses providing problem-solving treatment, after being trained for this purpose (see Chapter 5). Problem-solving is effective in enhancing the patient's sense of personal control and achievement, which are impaired in depression (see Figure 7.2 for a cognitive model of depression). Less severe depressive episodes may benefit from guided self-help or computerized CBT, neither of which requires specialist intervention. For patients who have had an episode of depression in the past, mindfulness-based cognitive therapy is effective in preventing further relapse (Teasdale et al 2000).

Medication as treatment for depression

Antidepressant medication is an effective treatment for depression. It is more likely to be considered as the optimal treatment when the depression is more severe or is recurrent. Care needs to be taken when deciding whether to start antidepressant medication in the physically ill. Considerations should include: the general health status of the individual, the potential side effects of the antidepressant, and the possible interactions with any other drugs the patient is taking.

The drugs of choice for treating depression in the physically ill are *selective serotonin reuptake inhibitors* (SSRIs). These drugs tend to have fewer side effects than other antidepressants, and two of them, Citalopram and Sertraline, have been identified as having fewer interactions with other drugs (NICE 2009).

Self-help resources

Books

Gilbert, P. (2009) *Overcoming Depression: A Self-help Guide using Cognitive Behavioural Techniques* (3rd edition) London: Robinson.

Greenberger, D. and Padesky, C. (1995) *Mind Over Mood: Change How You Feel by Changing the Way You Think.* London: Guilford Press.

Williams, M., Teasdale, J., Segal, Z. and Kabat-Zinn, J. (2007) *The Mindful Way Through Depression: Freeing Yourself from Chronic Unhappiness.* London: Guilford Press.

Internet

Depression Alliance: http://www.depressionalliance.org/help-and-information/self-help-coping.php

Mind: www.mind.org.uk/help/diagnoses_and_conditions/depression?

Moodjuice: http://www.moodjuice.scot.nhs.uk/depression.asp

Summary

Depression is often the most severe mental condition that will be encountered in nursing practice, so it is important to be able to recognize it and how to find treatment for the patient. Other less common but very severe conditions, the psychoses, will also be seen in practice, and these are the focus of the next chapter.

Key points

- Depression is a serious, distressing and disabling condition that is common in health care settings;
- Although there is some similarity to sadness and other reactions to life, depression has particular features that can be recognized in practice;
- There are screening tools that facilitate recognition and onward referral for specialist treatment;
- Depression is amenable to treatment by mental health specialists;
- Good nursing care can make a significant difference to the experience of the depressed patient in health care.

References

Bair, M.J., Robinson, R.L., Katon, W. and Kroenke, K. (2003) Depression and pain comorbidity: a literature review, *Archives of Internal Medicine*, 163 (10), 2433–2445.

Beck, A., Rush, A., Shaw, B. and Emery, G. (1979) *Cognitive Therapy of Depression*. New York: Guilford Press.

Brugha, T.S. (1993) Depression in the terminally ill, *British Journal of Hospital Medicine*, 50 (4), 175–181.

Chochinov, H.M., Wilson, K.G., Enns, M. and Lander, S. (1997) 'Are you depressed?' Screening for depression in the terminally ill, *American Journal of Psychiatry*, 154 (5), 674–676.

Cox, J., Holden, J. and Sagovsky, R. (1987) Detection of postnatal depression: development of the 10-item Edinburgh Postnatal Depression Scale, *British Journal of Psychiatry*, 150, 782–786.

Endicott, J. (1984) Measurement of depression in patients with cancer, *Cancer*, 53, 2243–2249.

Goldberg, D.P. and Bridges, K. (1988) Somatic presentations of psychiatric illness in primary care settings, *Journal of Psychosomatic Research*, 32 (2), 137–144.

Harvey, S., Hotopf, M., Overland, S. and Mykletun, A. (2010) Physical activity and common mental disorders, *British Journal of Psychiatry*, 197, 357–364.

Kroenke, K., Spitzer, R. and Williams, J. (2001) The PHQ-9: validity of a brief depression severity measure, *Journal of General Internal Medicine*, 16 (9), 606–613.

Moorey, S. and Greer, S. (2002) *Cognitive Behaviour Therapy for People with Cancer*. Oxford: Oxford University Press.

Moussavi, S., Chatterji, S., Verdes, E., Tandon, A., Patel, V. and Ustun, B. (2007) Depression, chronic diseases, and decrements in health: results from the World Health Surveys, *The Lancet*, 370 (9590), 808–809.

NICE (2009) *Depression in adults with a chronic physical health problem. NICE clinical guideline 91.* Available online at www.nice.org.uk/CG91.

Rayner, L., Higginson, I.J., Price, A. and Hotopf, M. (2010) *The Management of Depression in Palliative Care: European Clinical Guidelines.* London: Department of Palliative Care, Policy & Rehabilitation. (www.kcl.ac.uk/schools/medicine/depts/palliative)/European Palliative Care Research Collaborative (www.epcrc.org).

Roth, A., Kornblith, A., Batel-Copel, L. et al (1998) Rapid screening for psychologic distress in men with prostate carcinoma: a pilot study, *Cancer*, 82, 1904–1908.

Teasdale, J., Segal, Z., Williams, J., Ridgeway, V., Soulsby, J. and Lau, M. (2000) Prevention of relapse recurrence in major depression by mindfulness-based cognitive therapy, *Journal of Consulting and Clinical Psychology*, 68, 615–623.

Westbrook, D., Kennerley, H. and Kirk, J. (2011) *An Introduction to Cognitive Behaviour Therapy: Skills and Applications* (2nd edition). London: SAGE Publications.

Zigmond, A.S. and Snaith, R.P. (1983) The hospital anxiety and depression scale, *Acta Psychiatrica Scandinavica*, 67, 361–370.

8

WORKING WITH THE PSYCHOTIC PERSON AND WITH THE SERIOUSLY MENTALLY ILL

Learning objectives

By the end of this chapter, you should be able to:

- understand the personal experience of psychosis and its social impact;
- identify clinical features of psychotic conditions and serious mental illness;
- explore how sensitive and sympathetic nursing care helps people experiencing psychosis;
- understand the principles of consent and capacity and the applications of mental health law in caring for the psychotic patient;
- discuss effective management of psychotic conditions and confusional states, working with mental health services when necessary.

Introduction

Psychotic conditions are not commonly encountered in general adult nursing practice, but they can be perplexing or frightening when they are. Psychoses are usually described as functional, where diagnosis is based on symptoms and behaviour, but there is some overlap with confusional states which have organic causes. Much of the management of psychoses, particularly functional psychoses, is specialized, and is the remit of mental health professionals. However, it is important for the general adult nurse to have some understanding of these conditions, and they can have a positive role in providing sensitive and knowledgeable nursing care.

What do we mean by psychosis?

Psychosis is synonymous with the lay term *madness*. This conjures images of people out of control, 'going mad'. It has a sense of something 'other', different, dangerous. The medical term psychosis does refer to something very different from what most people would consider to be normal human experience. Acute psychosis is often disturbing, strange and frightening to the person who experiences it, as well as to those around them. However, there is a picture emerging of psychosis as not a single, alien, disturbed state, but rather a range of experiences, some of which would be familiar to most people. Psychosis can be seen, therefore, as the extreme end of a continuum of human experience.

There are two main types of psychotic experience: hallucinations and delusions. Hallucinations are a disorder of perception, and can involve any of the senses (see Box 8.1). They usually occur in serious mental illness, but they can also occur in organic states such as delirium, in bereavement, where the bereaved person believes they see or hear their lost loved one, and it is not uncommon for people to have auditory or visual hallucinations briefly when they are falling asleep (hypnagogic hallucinations) or waking up (hypnopompic hallucinations).

Many hallucinations in serious mental illness are very disturbing and disabling:

The voices were telling me how worthless I was and how nobody cared, and how pointless my existence was, and that I would be better off not on this earth. And, I thought, well, you know, nobody's listening to me so may be the voices are right…

I've had no respite for nearly 15 years of voices. And that's so wearing. That just grinds you down. And they are horrible. Some people's voices are mildly derogatory, mine are abusive and threatening. There are four men. I don't know who they are. I just know they are my voices, and they are just vile.

Ceridwen (available online at www.healthtalkonline.org/) © 2012 University of Oxford

However, it is important to recognize that not all auditory hallucinations are negative, and some people find their voices helpful or inspiring (see also Box 8.2):

And sometimes you get extremely kind voices as well. I got reminded to take my medication when I came out of hospital at one point. I was having difficulty, I didn't have a, a proper system for sorting out my medication, and I saw a friend of mine on the bus, and he was going up to the psychiatric unit to see some friends, and he was like, 'Oh hi. How you're doing?' I said, 'Yes, fine. But I keep forgetting to take my medication and that.' And I suppose that was half past one, two o'clock in the afternoon. Around came 5 o'clock and I got in my head the voice, 'medication', which was the call at the hospital at 5 o'clock for people to come and queue up for medication, you know, so, they can be, you know, that's a really practical salvation as well. But they can boost your confidence or whatever, you know.

Kirsty (available online at www.healthtalkonline.org/) © 2012 University of Oxford

---

Box 8.1 Types of hallucination

Auditory (hearing voices)   Auditory hallucinations are the most common in serious functional mental illness. They are usually experienced as another person talking inside the person's head. These may be experienced as threatening or abusive.

Visual   These are common in organic confusional states and may also occur in functional mental illness.

Tactile   These are usually experienced on or just below the skin, and may be felt to be creatures crawling or burrowing (this is associated with drug and alcohol use). Sometimes they are experienced more deeply inside the body.

Olfactory and gustatory   Experiencing, respectively, a smell or a perception of taste in the absence of a related external stimulus.

Delusions are a disorder of thought. They are described as beliefs that are held strongly by the person in spite of evidence to the contrary, and do not fit with common belief systems within their culture. Of course, many people hold beliefs that not everyone would agree with, and one person may present evidence that they feel disproves the beliefs of another. However, delusions have a different quality. They do not appear out of a process of logical argument, and they may have a basis in another psychotic experience like a hallucination. In serious mental illness, patients can experience a range of different types of delusions (see Box 8.3). Persecutory or paranoid delusions are a common distressing form of delusion, often associated with persecutory auditory hallucinations. Delusions can become a problem if they lead to extreme or dangerous forms of behaviour. For example, a person who believes they are being persecuted by the police may avoid going out and become socially isolated and neglect their basic needs. Or they may react by carrying a weapon for self-protection. Other disorders are of *thought possession*, where the person believes that their thoughts are being inserted, withdrawn or broadcast to others outside of their control.

The following is an example of a delusion of reference:

But like the other types of things that happened was I'd be watching the telly and my perception would be that what they were saying related to me...This is interesting. And like, you're like God, thank God I watched the telly. Thank God I watched that programme. It really enlightened me. So it's very subtle, but it's like your perception of reality is like a bit distorted. Because to any one else, it's like oh yeah I watched that TV programme. That was interesting. But to me, it's like oh God. It's heaven sent. Do you know what I mean. Yes. It's like that.

Jenni (available online at www.healthtalkonline.org/) © 2012 University of Oxford

---

Box 8.2 Hearing voices – always a problem?

There is evidence of people *hearing voices* throughout history, and they have often been interpreted as having spiritual meaning; for example, hearing the voice of God. In more recent times, with the rise of psychiatry, hearing voices in the absence of an external stimulus has been interpreted as auditory hallucinations, symptomatic of psychotic illness, particularly schizophrenia. However, there is now a widespread Hearing Voices Movement, which views hearing voices as a valid human experience, not psychopathology.

Romme and Escher (2000) suggest that there are compelling reasons to re-evaluate our understanding of hearing voices, and not see them solely as evidence of mental illness. These are:

- people who hear voices need to find acceptance for their experiences;
- some people are able to live successfully with their voices, without needing psychiatric help;
- conventional psychiatric treatments are not always effective and usually have side effects, so alternative approaches to management should be sought.

Hearing voices can be interpreted as a meaningful experience, linked to the individual's personal history, often based in or triggered by traumatic events. Viewed from this perspective, engaging with the voices can be helpful, and has the potential for healing and recovery, in a similar way to patients exploring their personal illness narrative.

Box 8.3 Common types of delusion

Persecutory   Persecutory or paranoid delusions are where a person believes they are threatened in some way by others, either a person or an organization, in the absence of adequate evidence. The threat can be perceived to be plotting to undermine their best interests (e.g. spying on them), or actual acts of aggression (e.g. a belief that a neighbour is poisoning them).

Grandiose   A belief that the person is special in an exaggerated or improbable way; for example, has special powers or is a member of a royal family. This is common in states of elevated mood or *mania*.

Reference   This is the belief that events in the outside world are connected to the person in a special way; for example, that items in the news refer directly to them or that major disasters have happened because of them.

Control   The person believes that their actions are directly controlled by an outside agency (though not the religious view that God controls our lives), and that they have a passive role in relation to their actions.

Guilt   Delusions of guilt are common in severe depression. The person feels that things they have done in the past are very bad and will have consequences for them or those close to them.

Somatic   These are strongly held beliefs that the person has a serious physical illness, in spite of evidence to the contrary.

What leads to a person receiving a diagnosis of psychosis?

If psychosis is at one end of a continuum of human experience, then what distinguishes someone who receives a diagnosis of psychotic illness from someone who does not? Mild degrees of psychotic experience, hearing things that others do not, are common in adolescents, possibly occurring in 20 per cent of the population (Murray and Jones 2012). Adolescence is a time of considerable personal change and stress, and teenagers also commonly experience anxiety, depression and suicidal thoughts. However, a minority of people who experience psychotic symptoms during this period go on to develop a psychotic illness, usually starting in early adulthood.

Hallucinations and delusions are not uncommon on the general population. In a major study of the incidence of psychotic experiences in the British adult population, after excluding people who already had a psychiatric diagnosis, 5.5 per cent were found to have experienced a psychotic symptom (i.e. hallucination or delusion) within the previous year (Johns et al 2004). This was found to be more common in people with anxiety and depression, drug dependence and a history of victimization (e.g. bullying, violence, sexual abuse). There was also an association between recent stressful life events and paranoid thoughts.

The ways in which these factors affect the development of psychotic illness (or vice versa) are not clear. There does appear to be a relationship between psychotic illness and anxiety and depression, and it is possible that if these conditions are not detected or effectively managed, some individuals go on to develop psychosis. On the other hand, it could be that the presence of anxiety and depression lessen the sense of personal control, so that people feel less able to manage their mental state. Drug and alcohol misuse may indicate problems with coping, and they may also be used to suppress psychotic experiences. The relationship with stress and victimization events is less clear. These events are likely to precipitate psychosis in some vulnerable individuals, but it is also possible that vulnerability leads to situations of risk or to the persecutory interpretation of events.

An active and positive approach to coping with problems and stressful life events may, then, afford some protection against psychotic episodes in vulnerable people. Active coping strategies, including problem-solving, help-seeking and distraction, are associated with a greater sense of control in the face of psychotic symptoms. However, a significant factor that determines the need for care is the extent to which an individual acts on psychotic delusions or hallucinations (Bak et al 2003). They are also more likely to become a psychiatric patient if their voices are negative (Romme and Escher 2000).

This is an account of what happened before a first diagnosis of psychosis:

And this was when I first went in psychosis. Basically I began to stop sleeping. And accompanying that I couldn't stop thinking and for the first time in years the thought of self-harm became really prominent in my mind again. And I told my wife that that was what I was thinking. And we went to see a GP who made an emergency referral to a psychologist who was going to see me quite quickly to see if we could do something about it...I began to think that...my blood had been poisoned by evil spirits and that I was evil, and that there were spirits around me, warping my thoughts and changing my thoughts, and that was very frightening and I didn't know what to do with it.

Graham (available online at www.healthtalkonline.org/) © 2012 University of Oxford

In this case, the person experiencing the psychosis knew something was wrong and sought help. In other cases, the person may be suspicious of others or afraid to ask for help, and only come to the attention of psychiatric services if their family or other members of the community take some action. This can be because their behaviour is frightening, strange or otherwise gives cause for concern.

Reflection point

Can you think of the most anxious or frightened that you have ever been? Do you remember what was going through your mind at the time? Do you recognize anything different about these thoughts and feelings from the ones that you usually experience?

Acute psychotic conditions

Acute psychotic episodes can occur in isolation, or as an acute crisis in the context of a serious long-term mental illness. Single isolated *brief psychotic episodes* can occur at times of severe stress, and this may occasionally be seen in the context of physical illness. Recovery is usually rapid and complete.

There are some other conditions that may present in a similar way to acute psychosis. *Mania* or *hypomania* is a state of elevated mood or euphoria, and a high level of energy and activity. There are sometimes psychotic features, like hallucinations and delusions that have a grandiose nature. Behaviour is often extreme and socially uninhibited, and can put the person at risk; for example, reckless driving, casual sexual relationships. Manic episodes often form part of a cycle of high and low moods in *bipolar affective disorder* (sometimes called *manic depressive psychosis*). *Dissociative disorders* can involve the temporary loss of memory, personal identity, sensation and/or physical function, in the absence of physical pathology and often related to trauma.

Serious mental illness (SMI)

SMI is a term used to describe the most severe, long-term and disabling mental health conditions, usually describing *schizophrenia* and *bipolar affective disorder*, though it can include other long-term conditions such as depression. SMI is distinctive in a number

---

Box 8.4 Features of schizophrenia

- *Hallucinations*: usually auditory
- *Delusions*, often of control or reference
- *Disturbance of thought possession*: thought insertion, withdrawal, broadcasting
- *Disruption of thinking*, disorganized speech
- *Negative and passive behaviour*: apathy, emotional response limited or inappropriate
- *Social withdrawal*, loss of interest and social engagement, sometimes self-neglect

of ways: the symptom experience tends to be severe and distressing, the course of the illness may fluctuate but is long term, treatments can cause additional problems and there are social effects secondary to the illness itself.

Schizophrenia is a well-established diagnostic category but it has always been problematic and controversial. It is more accurate to say that it covers a range of psychological conditions rather than being a single diagnosis. The primary features of schizophrenia are hallucinations and delusions, disturbance of thought possession, disruption to thinking and communication, and features of negative and passive behaviour, including social withdrawal (see Box 8.4). The following is a personal account of schizophrenia that illustrates the interaction between an olfactory hallucination and a persecutory delusion:

> Like once I went to visit my friends and when I got home, all I could smell of was cats litter. And like it stank. And I was like how the hell has this happened, I didn't even go near their cat litter. And I was like, oh my God, they've cursed me. Do you know what I mean. Just imagine, imagine that in your reality. Like, it's like, what on earth? But that was like it was liked they cursed me when I went to visit them. They must be witches and stuff like that. It was really bizarre. Yes. Really interesting. I don't know what that was about or, yes, but I know now looking back, like my experiences, my subconscious was like coming into the front of my brain. So like, weird thoughts that I had, like I think I built up a weird perception of myself, and a weird perception of the world, and then it all exploded, because it got too much. Do you know what I mean?

Jenni (available online at www.healthtalkonline.org/) © 2012 University of Oxford

Bipolar affective disorder is characterized by recurrent episodes of mania or hypomania and depression (see Box 8.5). In contrast, depression without mania is a *unipolar affective disorder*; that is, a mood disorder of only one mood type. There is also a condition that involves episodes of mixed mood and psychotic disturbance termed *schizoaffective disorder.*

Box 8.5 Features of bipolar affective disorder

Mania is characterized by:

- elevated mood or elation;
- increased energy and activity;
- decreased need for sleep;
- loss of attention and distractibility, racing thoughts;
- grandiose ideas;
- loss of social inhibitions;
- extravagant and extreme behaviour;
- in some cases, psychotic features (hallucinations and delusions) are also present.

Hypomania is a less severe form of elevated mood. Unlike mania, it does not cause serious disruption to social or occupational functioning, and it does not have psychotic features.

Depression is a feature of bipolar disorder, and depressive episodes are more common than manic ones.

Physical health effects of SMI

People with SMI have a number of risk factors for physical health problems. This is partly because of the effects of the illness itself, but also treatment effects, self-harming behaviours, including use of non-prescribed drugs, and the social impacts of serious illness (see Box 8.6). Schizophrenia is associated with a number of physical health problems, including cardiovascular and respiratory disease, obesity, diabetes mellitus, some cancers, infections and reduced mortality (Pack 2009).

Box 8.6 Physical effects of SMI

- *Effects of mental illness*: lack of sleep, rest and relaxation
- *Self-neglect*: poor diet, weight loss or obesity, dehydration, poor hygiene
- *Apathy*: lack of exercise and activity
- *Use of drugs*: tobacco-related respiratory problems, effects of alcohol or non-prescribed drugs
- *Effects of medication*: extrapyramidal side effects
- *Self-harm*: self-injury, effects of overdose or other self-harming acts or behaviours
- *Infections*: reduced immunity, exposure to infective agents (e.g. sexually transmitted infections)
- *Effects of social deprivation*: poor housing and general amenities

---

Social effects of SMI

SMI has considerable social effects (see Box 8.7). Because of the nature of psychosis, it is difficult to articulate the experience, and this can leave the individual feeling isolated. Those most sympathetic are likely to be professionals or other people with psychosis, thereby narrowing the person's social network. They may also experience prejudice and discrimination, excluding them from social contact, employment and housing. These factors can combine to result in the *social exclusion* of the person; that is, they become unable to fully engage with their community, and exist only on the margins of society.

They think that it's just that I'm lazy and that I don't want to do nothing and that I should get out and do things for myself like go back to work...and that because they see me as an intelligent person but they don't see things behind, it's just they can't see the mental, where if you've got a broken arm you can see that you've got an injury, you know, with mental health they can't see it…I haven't been able to work because I can't, I don't stay well for more than six weeks…I was a nurse before I became unwell…It's very, I feel isolated because I had friends in work, all my friends were in work in London and I've got no friends really that are down here that I worked with, it's all friends from the mental health services.

Ugo (available online at www.healthtalkonline.org/) © 2012 University of Oxford

There remains social *stigma* attached to mental illness. Stigma is described as damaged or spoiled social identity, and it can be attached to someone on the basis of looking or behaving differently. Unpredictability of behaviour, and admissions for psychiatric treatment, can contribute to the attribution of stigma in the mentally ill. Health professionals can also stigmatize the mentally ill if they do not treat them in a respectful or sympathetic manner.

Box 8.7 Social effects of SMI

- Disrupted relationships
- Social isolation
- Disruption or loss of employment
- Loss of income (excessive spending in manic episodes)
- Housing problems
- Social exclusion
- Social stigma

The management of SMI

There are a number of treatment approaches used in the management of SMI. Although drug treatments are the most common, they have limitations, both in terms of their success, and in the significant side effects associated with them. There is a widely acknowledged role for social and interpersonal therapies, which not only avoid these side effects, but often mitigate the social isolation that is commonly encountered in SMI.

Antipsychotic medication

Antipsychotic medication is commonly used to treat both schizophrenia and manic episodes. This is generally divided into two types. Typical antipsychotic drugs include chlorpromazine, flupenthixol and haloperidol. These have been in use for a long period of time, so have proven effectiveness in suppressing psychotic symptoms, but they have many side effects. Atypical antipsychotics, such as clozapine, olanzapine and risperidone, are more recently introduced drugs that have fewer extrapyramidal side effects (see Box 8.8). Antipsychotics are usually given in tablet form but can also be given as depot injections, which release the drug slowly.

Box 8.8 Side effects of antipsychotic medication

Antidopaminergic or extrapyramidal side effects are:
- dystonia, painful spasms of muscles, especially in the neck and face;
- akathisia, a distressing feeling of restless;
- Parkinsonian symptoms, tremor, muscle stiffness, shuffling gait;
- tardive dyskinesia, involuntary muscular movements associated with longer-term antipsychotic use.

Anticholinergic side effects are:
- dry mouth;
- blurred vision;
- constipation.

Note: This is not an exhaustive list. See the *British National Formulary* for details of specific drug side effects and drug interactions.

Mood stabilizing medication

Mood stabilizing medication is used in the longer-term management of bipolar disorder, and includes lithium carbonate, sodium valproate and carbamazepine. All of these drugs have side effects but particular care needs to be taken with lithium. Blood lithium levels have to be monitored regularly to ensure that they are within the therapeutic range but do not reach a level of toxicity, which if not detected can be fatal.

Social

Social or psychosocial approaches to managing schizophrenia focus on psychoeducation (psychological health education), social support, involving the family and other carers, and maintaining independence. These are often undertaken in the community by a multiprofessional mental health team, to reduce hospital admissions and minimize social exclusion.

Cognitive behavioural therapy

CBT can be used in the management of schizophrenia and has also been used to treat bipolar disorder. In schizophrenia, CBT focuses on the following process: engagement and assessment, developing coping strategies, understanding psychosis, working with beliefs underlying delusions and hallucinations, addressing emotional reactions and managing social disability (Garety et al 2000).

Working with voices

There are a number of approaches to helping people to engage with their voices with the intention of reducing the distress associated with them, rather than suppressing them (Romme and Escher 2000). Kingdon and Turkington (2004) describe treatment based on the principle that it is anxiety and powerlessness that make voices distressing and problematic. They explore other ways of interpreting voices, as a 'normal' response to trauma or abuse, for example. Another technique involves engaging in a dialogue with the voices, and exploring their personal meaning for the individual. Davies et al (1999) suggest that voices have a pragmatic function or purpose for the hearer. By engaging in a dialogue with their voices, as a form of personal narrative, their meaning can be uncovered, and a new, more constructive relationship negotiated with them. This can also be explored within a group setting (Martin 2000).

Assessment of psychosis

The assessment of a patient's mental state is specialized and should be undertaken by a psychiatrist or other mental health professional. However, it is important for the general nurse to have an understanding of what this involves, and to recognize the main symptoms of psychotic illness. Mental state examination is the standard approach used in psychiatry (Box 8.9). Physical causes of mental disturbance should always be considered in assessment. These include any drugs, prescribed or otherwise, that the patient may have taken.

Box 8.9 Mental state examination

Attention and level of consciousness	• Ability to pay attention to what is said and to the surroundings
	• Level of consciousness: from clear, to clouded, to coma
Appearance and behaviour	• Facial expression, eye contact. Presentation, including clothing (any sign that the patent is not taking care of themselves?)
	• Body posture, movements, gestures
	• Activity: restlessness, agitation, withdrawal
Mood (affect)	• Examples: anxiety, depression, fear, anger, suspicion, euphoria, hopelessness. Ask about suicidal ideas
Speech	• Form: is the speech clear and coherent?
	• Is there pressure of speech (found in mania) or is speech retarded (depression)?
	• Is the pitch and volume appropriate to the circumstances?
	• Content: does the patient talk about anything bizarre or seemingly irrelevant to the conversation?

Thoughts	• Form: does the patient believe their thoughts are controlled in any way (thought possession)? Are any of their ideas markedly strange or worrying (delusional)?
	• Content: for example, guilt, persecution/paranoia, ideas of reference
Perceptions	• Illusions (misinterpretations of actual stimuli), hallucinations (experiences in the absence of external stimuli)
Cognitive state	• Orientation in time, place and person
	• Concentration
	• Any disruption of recent or long-term memory
Understanding and rapport	• Understanding of the nature of the illness or problem
	• Quality and strength of relationship with assessor

Nursing care of psychotic states

- *Engagement*   *Accepting* the patient and their experience of psychosis is a first step towards engagement with them. It is also very important to include the family and other carers in assessment and the process of care. Carers may be distressed or frightened by the patient's experience, and it can be extremely valuable for the nurse and carers to spend time *being with* the patient, providing a calming and comforting personal presence.

- *Clear communication*   This is particularly important if the patient is psychotic as there is the potential for misunderstandings. Distress and anger can make it more difficult to communicate in an empathic way. It is important to check for understanding at each stage of communication.

- *Assessment*   The nurse should aim to identify the nature of the patient's experience and take initial steps towards a full mental state examination as soon as mental health professionals can be involved.

- *Maintain a safe environment*   People experiencing psychosis may act impulsively or unpredictably. They can pose a risk to themselves or others as they respond to mental experiences that may be threatening or controlling. It may be necessary to get additional staff to contain the situation, and to refer to local policies on the management of difficult or challenging behaviour (see Chapter 9). Tranquilizing medication can be used under these circumstances, but psychiatric advice should be taken first. Great caution needs to be taken to ensure the patient's civil liberties are respected. The patient's physical health should remain an area of concern during psychotic episodes; for example, ensuring adequate hydration and nutrition.

- *Teamwork and onward referral*   Working together as a team ensures effective decision-making and is supportive for all of the individuals involved. Referral to a psychiatric team should be made as soon as possible.

Nursing care of SMI

People with a SMI will be admitted to hospital at times with physical health problems, and much of their management will be undertaken in the primary care setting. In dealing with SMI, all of the aspects of nursing care given above are important. In addition, the following should be given attention.

Maintain physical health Self-neglect is common in SMI, so nurses should always support and encourage adequate diet, exercise and hygiene. Care should also be taken to assess for comorbid conditions, drug and alcohol use.

Manage medication side effects Antipsychotic and mood-stabilizing drugs have a number of potentially serious side effects that should be monitored.

Social support and support to the family helps to maximize the patient's personal and social identity and minimize the effects of social exclusion.

Confusional states

The confusional states are conditions where a clear physical cause can be identified for severe psychological disturbance. These can be further divided into acute and chronic states. Acute organic confusion is usually referred to as *delirium*, though it can also be termed *acute confusional state*. The problem with the latter term is that confusion is also a symptom, characterized by disorganized thinking or uncharacteristic, strange behaviour. Delirium is therefore a better term to use for the condition to avoid this ambiguity (Schuurmans et al 2001). A chronic confusional state is better termed *dementia*. The differences between delirium and dementia are given in Box 8.10.

Box 8.10 Delirium and dementia		
Symptoms	**Delirium**	**Dementia**
Onset	Acute (hours to days)	Chronic (months to years)
Course	Usually reversible	Progressive
Level of consciousness	Clouded, reduced awareness of environment	Clear
Cognition	Disorganized thinking, disorientation, impaired memory for recent events	Disturbed thinking and reasoning, disorientation, impaired memory for recent events
Variation during the day	Worse in the evening, disturbed sleep/wake cycle	No fluctuation
Emotions	Distressed, anxious, fearful, suspicious, sometimes apathetic	Emotionally labile, or apathetic and irritable, may become disinhibited
Hallucinations and delusions	Often present – delusions usually transient	Sometimes present
Activity	Agitated and restless or inactive	Usually normal

Delirium can be caused by any factor or agent that disturbs neurological function. The list of potential causes is therefore almost limitless (Box 8.11 gives a range of potential causes). Delirium is most common in the older patient, but can occur at any age. Vulnerability to delirium varies between individuals. For the person experiencing it, delirium can evoke fear, anxiety, helplessness, loneliness and bewilderment (Schuurmans et al 2001). It is important to recognize and manage delirium effectively: it is a serious life-threatening condition and mortality associated with delirium is very high.

Box 8.11 Causes of delirium	
Drugs	Any drug – alcohol, opiates, antipsychotics, lithium, benzodiazepines, corticosteroids, recreational drugs, drug or alcohol withdrawal
Infections	Septicaemia, encephalitis, urinary tract infection, chest infection
Metabolic	Dehydration, electrolyte imbalance, hypoxia, renal failure, cardiac failure, hepatic failure
Neurological	Head injury, cerebrovascular accident, epilepsy, space-occupying lesions
Endocrine	Diabetic crises – hyperglycaemia, hypoglycaemia; hyperthyroidism, hypothyroidism
Environmental	Sensory deprivation or overstimulation, sleep disturbance, change of routine or place of residence, hospitalization, hearing or visual problems
Other	Constipation, urinary retention, post-operative recovery, stay in intensive care

Assessment

A thorough assessment should always be taken to confirm the diagnosis of delirium. This should include the use of terminology that describes behaviour rather than simply states that the patient is confused (Schuurmans et al 2001).

Assessment tools include:

- Mini Mental State Examination (MMSE) (Folstein et al 1975)
- Confusion Assessment Method (CAM) (Inouye et al 1990)

Nursing care of delirium and dementia

- Identify and manage any causal or contributory factors
- Provide good nursing care, but keeping interventions to the minimum

- Keep all communication clear, brief and to the point (ensure patient has hearing aids and glasses if needed)
- Optimize sensory input and orientation: reduce unnecessary noise or changes to the patient's environment, provide regular cues to the time of day
- Respond to hallucinations or illusions with explanations where possible
- Ensure the safety of the acutely disturbed patient, but avoid the use of restraint
- Keep medication use to the minimum necessary

Consent and capacity

Given the range of mental disturbance that can be encountered in mental disorders, it is important to be familiar with the legal framework for ensuring consent to treatment, whether this is for physical or for mental health problems. There are two main legal statutes that are relevant to this area in England and Wales: the Mental Capacity Act 2005 and the Mental Health Act 1983. In addition, *common law* is relevant under certain circumstances, particularly emergencies.

The Mental Capacity Act 2005

This act makes provision for decisions to be made on behalf of patients if they lack capacity, that is, the ability to make decisions, on the basis of a disturbance or impairment of mental function. The law assumes that everyone has capacity unless they are judged to lack it. This decision cannot be simply because they make an unwise decision, or on the basis of their age, appearance, condition or behaviour alone. Incapacity means the patient is unable to:

- understand information relevant to the decision, including the consequences of their decision or of not making a decision;
- retain the information for long enough to make a decision;
- use the information to make a decision; or
- communicate their decision.

If the patient lacks capacity, staff may delay a decision if the patient's condition is likely to improve, or, after consultation with family or other carers, make a treatment decision in the patient's best interests. Being mentally ill does not by itself mean that a patient lacks capacity. For example, a patient may require compulsory treatment for psychosis but have the capacity to refuse treatment for a physical condition, even if their decision appears not to be in their best interests.

In Scotland, the equivalent legislation is the Adults with Incapacity (Scotland) Act 2000:

www.legislation.gov.uk/asp/2000/4/contents

In Northern Ireland, there is currently no specific legislation on capacity, so cases are dealt with under case law, general legislation and guidance from the Department of Health, Social Services and Public Safety. A joint mental health and mental capacity act for Northern Ireland is in preparation.

The Mental Health Act 1983

The act makes provision, in England and Wales, for compulsory detention in hospital of an individual, because of the nature or degree of their mental disorder, for assessment and/or treatment, if they are deemed to be a risk to themselves or others. There are two main sections of the act dealing with detention to a psychiatric hospital (or a psychiatric unit in a general hospital):

- **Section 2** covers detention for assessment (in some cases followed by treatment) for up to 28 days.
- **Section 3** covers detention for treatment, if this can only be delivered in hospital, for up to six months.

Treatment can be for drug or alcohol dependence if this is an appropriate part of treating the mental disorder. The act only deals with mental disorder, so it cannot be used to treat physical illness. However, it can include actions dealing with the physical state of the patient if this is necessary to treat the mental disorder. This could include, for example, taking blood samples to monitor the patient's reaction to antipsychotic drugs. *Section 5(2)* can potentially be used in the general hospital to detain a patient for up to 72 hours for assessment of their mental state.

In Scotland, the equivalent legislation is the Mental Health (Care and Treatment) (Scotland) Act 2003:

www.legislation.gov.uk/asp/2003/13/contents

In Northern Ireland, the relevant legislation is the Mental Health (Northern Ireland) Order 1986:

www.legislation.gov.uk/nisi/1986/595

Working with mental health services

The general nurse will inevitably work alongside mental health professionals in the care of people with psychotic conditions. In the community, this can include:

- *community mental health teams*, generic psychiatric services usually attached to a geographical area;
- *crisis resolution and home treatment teams*, with a focus on keeping SMI patients at home;
- *assertive outreach teams*, which provide services for people with severe and complex needs, often bridging both physical and mental health.

In the general hospital, psychiatric services are provided by *mental health liaison* or *liaison psychiatry* services:

In any of the above services, the main personnel will be:

- psychiatrists: doctors specializing in the management of mental illness;
- nurses: community psychiatric nurses, community specialists, and mental health liaison nurses, who work at the interface between mental and physical care;
- psychologists, usually clinical psychologists or health psychologists;
- some staff from these disciplines will be trained as psychotherapists.

Reflection point

Do you have experience of working with patients who have psychotic conditions or confusional states? Is there anything different that you would do now?

Summary

Psychotic conditions expose us to a range of extreme human experiences, which many nurses will feel fall outside of their expertise, but which can nonetheless be helped by sensitive and well-informed nursing care. The final chapter explores a range of behaviours that provide difficulties and challenges to nursing care.

Key points

- Psychosis is an extreme form of human experience, that can very distressing but that can also have personal meaning;
- Psychotic illness is characterized by hallucinations, often in the form of hearing voices, and delusions, a disorder of thought;
- SMIs are severe, disabling, long-term conditions, which have physical and social impacts and require specialist interventions and services;
- Organic confusional states are frequently encountered in hospitals;
- There are specific laws relating to consent to mental and physical treatments.

References

Bak, M., Myin-Germeys, I., Hanssen, M., Bijl, R., Vllebergh, W., Delespaul, P. and van Os, J. (2003) When does experience of psychosis result in a need for care? A prospective general population study, *Schizophrenia Bulletin*, 29 (2), 349–358.

Davies, P., Thomas, P. and Leudar, I. (1999) Dialogical engagement with voices: a single case study, *British Journal of Medical Psychology*, 72, 179–187.

Folstein, M., Folstein, S. and McHugh, P. (1975) Mini Mental State: a practical method for grading the cognitive state of patients for the clinician, *Journal of Psychiatric Research*, 12 (3), 189–198.

Garety, P., Fowler, D. and Kuipers, E. (2000) Cognitive-behavioral therapy for medication-resistant symptoms, *Schizophrenia Bulletin*, 26 (1), 73–86.

Inouye, S., van Dyck, C., Alessi, C., Balkin, S., Siegal, A. and Horwitz, R. (1990) Clarifying confusion: the Confusion Assessment Method, *Annals of Internal Medicine*, 113, 941–948.

Johns, L., Cannon, M., Singleton, N., Murray, R., Farrell, M., Brugha, T., Bebbington, P., Jenkins, R. and Meltzer, H. (2004) Prevalence and correlates of self-reported psychotic symptoms in the British population, *British Journal of Psychiatry*, 185, 298–305.

Kingdon, D. and Turkington, D. (2004) *Cognitive Therapy of Schizophrenia*. New York: Guilford Press.

Martin, P. (2000) Hearing voices and listening to those that hear them, *Journal of Psychiatric and Mental Health Nursing*, 7 (2), 135–141.

Murray, G. and Jones, P. (2012) Psychotic symptoms in young people without psychotic illness: mechanisms and meaning, *British Journal of Psychiatry*, 201, 4–6.

Pack, S. (2009) Poor physical health and mortality in patients with schizophrenia, *Nursing Standard*, 23 (21), 41–45.

Romme, M. and Escher, S. (2000) *Making Sense of Voices*. London: Mind Publications.

Schuurmans, M., Duursma, S. and Shortridge-Baggett, L. (2001) Early recognition of delirium: review of the literature, *Journal of Clinical Nursing*, 10, 721–729.

Further reading/resources

Burton, N. (2010) *Psychiatry* (2nd edition). Chichester: Wiley-Blackwell.

Maden, A. and Spencer-Lane, T. (2010) *Essential Mental Health Law: A Guide to the revised Mental Health Act and the Mental Capacity Act 2005*. London: Hammersmith Press.

Nash, M. (2010) *Physical Health and Well-being in Mental Health Nursing: Clinical Skills for Practice*. Maidenhead: Open University Press.

Regel, S. and Roberts, D. (eds) (2002) *Mental Health Liaison. A Handbook for Nurses and Health Professionals*. London: Baillière-Tindall.

Healthtalkonline experiences of psychosis: www.healthtalkonline.org/mental_health/experiences_of_psychosis

Hearing Voices Network England: www.hearing-voices.org/

9

WORKING WITH PEOPLE WHO PRESENT DIFFICULT BEHAVIOURS

Learning outcomes

By the end of this chapter, you should be able to:

- recognize which factors in the interaction with patients contribute to the perception that they are difficult to work with;
- understand the principles of managing challenging behaviours, aggression and violence and self-harm;
- identify the health effects of alcohol and drug misuse and dependence;
- understand how engagement and a non-judgemental approach to nursing care help people with drug and alcohol problems;
- discuss the effective nursing management of people who misuse alcohol and drugs, liaising with specialist services.

Introduction

There are various factors in the patient, and the interactions that nurses have with them, which can lead to the perception that they are difficult to work with. Challenging behaviours, including violence and aggression, can be difficult to manage in health care settings, so nurses need a knowledgeable and skilled approach to their management. Self-harm and suicidal behaviours are also difficult to work with, as they challenge our expectations about health-related behaviour. People who misuse alcohol and drugs form a group with significant health problems who benefit from effective management and nursing care.

The 'difficult patient'

We will inevitably like some patients and find it harder to nurse some patients than others. Stockwell's (1972) research into nurse–patient interaction on four hospital wards identified that there were factors in both the patient and nurse that led to patients being viewed as 'unpopular'. This included the degree of good humour and optimism that the patient displayed, and also the perception of the nurse about the quality of their communication and how suitable they were for the nursing care they provided. Patients who do not seem to fit with the social expectations of nurses, who are seen as demanding or ungrateful, for example, may meet with disapproval, stigma or social judgement (Johnson and Webb 1995).

Nurses may also feel uncomfortable nursing patients if their condition is unfamiliar, or they feel it does not fit with the ward environment or with their level of confidence or skills. In emergency departments, nurses may lack confidence in working with people who self-harm, or feel they are not equipped to meet their needs (McAllister et al 2002). People with mental health problems on general wards can be perceived as difficult or hard to help (Stockwell 1972), and people who cannot communicate their needs effectively can be perceived to be difficult and challenging to nurse (see Box 9.1) (Stokes 2000).

There are also groups of patients whose problems can alienate the people who work with them. The diagnosis of *personality disorder* is based on the personal experiences and behaviour of the individual. People with *borderline personality disorder*, for example, experience very intense and changeable moods, problems of self-identity, often feeling empty or abandoned, which can make them extremely sensitive to the way that others react to them. It is associated with feelings of dissociation and acts of self-harm, which can become a recurrent pattern of behaviour. These patients sometimes report unsympathetic attitudes among emergency department staff, though this is not always the case, and education helps to develop positive attitudes to their care (Commons Treloar and Lewis 2008).

Working with the difficult patient can present the nurse with challenges to engagement and empathy. Given the emotional intimacy that is evoked in situations of caring, both nurse and patient can feel uncomfortable if their needs or expectations are not met. Patients expect to be treated with care and concern, so they may feel excluded if they are treated with emotional coldness, if the nurse does not spend time with them or avoids eye contact (Shattell 2004). On their part, nurses need to interpret the needs of the patient with knowledge and understanding, and respond to them with compassion and respect.

Box 9.1 Factors that may make a patient 'difficult'

- They appear ungrateful or demanding, or do not meet expectations of how a patient should behave
- Their behaviour is challenging or aggressive
- The patient appears to disregard their own health or safety
- They have difficulties communicating their needs
- They evoke uncomfortable feelings in the nurse
- Their needs are hard to meet because of a lack of nursing skills, knowledge or resources
- The nurse lacks confidence in their management

Challenging behaviours

The term *challenging behaviour* has been used particularly in the context of mental health and learning disability nursing, and in the care of dementia. It includes behaviours that are aggressive or violent, offensive or disturbed, or are in other ways difficult to manage. It is a useful term in that it attributes the problem to the behaviour, not the patient (the behaviour is not always intentional), and it identifies that the problem is one of management. There are a number of potential causes of challenging behaviour (Box 9.2).

Box 9.2 Causes of challenging behaviour

- Anger or frustration
- Fear or anxiety
- Pain
- Intoxication with drugs or alcohol
- Confusion: delirium or dementia
- Acute mental disorder (e.g. mania, psychosis)
- Learning disability

Managing challenging behaviours

Challenging behaviours have a range of different presentations and causes. For example, single episodes of disturbed behaviour in the emergency department will present very differently from the long-term behavioural problems encountered in a nursing home with people who have dementia. However, there are some general management principles that apply in any situation:

- Communicate calmly and professionally, and as clearly as possible.
- Set limits on any behaviour that is not acceptable.
- Identify the cause of the behaviour or trigger event if this can be identified.
- Aim to resolve the problem if it is resolvable.

Violence and aggression

Violent and aggressive behaviour towards health care staff is surprisingly common. Numerous studies have shown that almost all hospital nurses experience violence or aggression at some point during their career, and the majority experience it on average once a month (O'Connell et al 2000; Hahn et al 2010). The most frequent form of violence is verbal, but physical assaults also occur. Violence is most often from patients and relatives, but aggression in the form of verbal abuse or intimidation is not uncommon from other members of staff (O'Connell et al 2000; Hahn et al 2010). Acts of aggression and violence may take place in any hospital department, most commonly medical and surgical wards, emergency departments and intensive care. In emergency departments, an assessment model has been devised to help nurses recognize behaviour that precedes acts of violence, STAMP (see Box 9.3).

Box 9.3 STAMP model for anticipating violence

- *Staring*: prolonged eye contact or avoidance of eye contact
- *Tone and volume of voice*: sharp, sarcastic or demeaning tone, increased volume
- *Anxiety*: for example, rapid speech, hyperventilation, disorientation
- *Mumbling*: incoherent speech, muttering
- *Pacing*: walking around bedroom or nurses' area

(Luck et al 2007)

Acts of aggression are also commonly reported in nursing homes, particularly involving patients with dementia. These can involve hitting, scratching, pulling, kicking or screaming. The causes of aggression or challenging behaviour in dementia are usually linked to cognitive impairments (Dettmore et al 2009). These make it more difficult for the patient to identify and communicate their needs, leading to frustration. Prevention and management of aggression therefore needs to focus on anticipating and meeting physical and psychological needs. These can include hunger, thirst, constipation, pain, light, noise, loneliness or insufficient help with daily living activities (Dettmore et al 2009).

Managing aggression and violence

Along with other forms of challenging behaviour, a calm and professional response is the first principle in managing aggression and violence. This is helped if the nurse has had suitable training and is familiar with the local policy on managing challenging situations. It is always important to identify a cause and/or trigger event in any challenging situation. In addition, the following are important aspects of management:

- *Maintain safety and manage the environment.* This can include moving vulnerable patients out of the immediate area, and keeping only key staff in the vicinity of the patient who is causing the disturbance.

- *Respond to the behaviour and set limits.* If the patient is causing distress or fear, it is a good idea to state this clearly to the patient. They may be feeling frightened and threatened themselves, and not realize the effect of their behaviour on other people. This can help them to take control of their behaviour and accept responsibility for it.

- *Respond to the person.* Show an empathic response if this is possible. Try to identify their emotions and respond to how they are feeling.

- *Resolve the situation as quickly as possible.* Allow sufficient time for the patient to feel that their concerns have been heard, but move on to solving problems as quickly as possible.

- *Use restraint only when it is unavoidable* and there are adequate numbers of suitably trained people to support this. Work as a team and involve additional expertise; for example, from a mental health team, if this is possible.

Self-care following aggression or violence

Aggression and violence leave staff with very uncomfortable feelings. Anger, fear and anxiety are common. If the nurse is not familiar with the range of situations that can provoke an incident, they may feel personally responsible, experiencing guilt, self-blame and shame, no matter how they dealt with the situation. Some nurses also experience symptoms of post-traumatic stress disorder (Needham et al 2005). This can have a demoralizing effect on nurses, so it is very important to prevent aggression and violence whenever possible. After a violent incident, staff should have the opportunity to talk the situation through in a *critical incident debriefing* session (Regel 2002). This provides the setting both to release difficult emotions and to discuss any lessons learned from the incident.

Case study: challenging behaviour

John Hancock is a young man in his twenties who has a severe learning disability. He usually lives in supported accommodation and has been admitted to hospital for assessment following an accident at his home. On admission, the ward staff have been given some written information on the nature of John's problems and the importance of clear communication when working with him. His key worker on the ward, Debbie, has taken time to explain what is going to happen to him while he is in hospital. He does not seem to respond verbally to this, so the nurse is not sure how much John has taken in. On the second day in hospital, he throws a chair across the bedroom. Debbie does not understand why this has happened, and is concerned that other patients on the ward will become frightened of him. Although she is worried how he will respond, she approaches him and tries to present a calm but concerned appearance, engaging him in direct eye contact. She says to John that she thinks he must be feeling scared and asks if John would come to the quiet room with her to talk about what has happened. John seems reluctant, but she offers her hand and he takes it. She sits him in a seat opposite the door and takes one next to it, but leaves the door open as she is not sure yet how he will react. She says that she would like to know why he became distressed, and explains that throwing a chair will upset the other patients, so he should not do that again. He says he wants to go home and he doesn't know why he is in hospital. Debbie decides she will need to spend more time with him to be sure that he understands what is going on. She finds the Hospital Communication Book (a resource for supporting people with learning disabilities in hospital) online at www.cuh.org.uk/resources/pdf/patient_information_leaflets/communication_guide/hospital_communication_book_section1.pdf and this gives her some ideas about the most effective ways to communication with John, including the use of gestures, pictures and symbols. Debbie shares this information with her colleagues on the ward.

Reflection point

Which aspects of communication were most important in Debbie's response to John's challenging behaviour?

Self-harm

Self-harm can mean a range of different behaviours. These include acts of self-poisoning or overdosing, self-cutting or burning. It is a more accurate term than *attempted suicide* or *parasuicide* as not all people who self-harm want to die. Acts of self-harm lead to about 150,000 emergency department attendances per annum in the United Kingdom, and nearly 70,000 admissions to hospital (NICE 2004). This does not represent the true extent of the problem, however, as many people do not attend hospital. People who self-harm commonly have problems in relationships, difficulties problem-solving, mental health problems, particularly schizophrenia and depression, alcohol misuse or a history of childhood sexual abuse (NICE 2004).

Self-poisoning usually involves taking tablets, most commonly paracetamol in the United Kingdom. As most acts of self-harm are impulsive, not planned, people tend to take what they have available to them at home. Most people who take overdoses are going through a personal crisis, and common feelings at the time are wanting to communicate how they feel to someone, wanting to get out of an overwhelming situation or to get help (Hjelmeland et al 2002). Self-poisoning is twice as common among females as males, and more common in adolescence and young adulthood. The majority of people who self-poison do not want to die, though there is a significant minority who do. Many people who self-poison also self-injure.

Self-injury is the deliberate act of damaging tissue, usually by cutting or burning, whilst in a distressed state of mind. This is not usually associated with suicidal intention, though some other acts of self-injury like hanging or self-shooting are. Self-injury often becomes a means of coping for people who experience very high levels of anxiety, associated with feelings of dissociation or depersonalization. A razor blade is the most common means used. There is a strong association between self-injury and eating disorders (Svirko and Hawton 2007). People who self-injure are seen less often in emergency departments than those who self-poison, and it is less likely that they will be offered follow-up treatment (Horrocks et al 2003).

The management of self-harm

Many people who self-harm do not present themselves at hospital, but seek help from family, friends, professionals, such as a counsellor or mental health team, or are seen in primary care. Whatever the setting, a professional response to an act of self-harm should consider the following:

- urgent assessment of the patient's physical condition and level of risk;
- prompt treatment of the patient's physical condition;

- psychosocial assessment as early as possible, making an onward referral to mental health services if necessary.

As in any emergency situation, *engagement* with the patient is very important. Patients have reported that they have better experiences of care after self-harm if they are provided with information about what is going on and if staff are sympathetic in their attitude. Those who have bad experiences can feel that they are treated with a lack of respect, treated differently from other patients, or that their psychological needs are ignored in favour of their physical needs (Taylor et al 2009). The NICE guidance (2004) on self-harm recommends that patients should be treated with respect and understanding, given full information about the management options available and involved in making decisions about their care.

The emergency department is the usual place of hospital attendance for people after self-harm. In addition to the care of the patient's physical state, it is essential that a psychosocial assessment is undertaken as soon as possible. How this is carried out varies considerably. In many hospitals, the emergency staff themselves carry out an initial assessment. Each emergency department should then have access to a mental health team that they can refer patients on to. Some hospitals have a dedicated self-harm team, either working alone or as part of a hospital-based mental health liaison service (NICE 2004). In many cases this team will comprise mental health nurses who specialize in the assessment and care of self-harm. Their assessment will focus on both critical elements like mental state and suicide risk, and therapeutic elements that aid personal control and coping, and this may form the basis of outpatient follow-up (Roberts and Mackay 1999). Assessment needs to take account of factors that contribute to repeated self-harm (Box 9.4) or suicide (Box 9.6).

Box 9.4 Risk factors for repetition of self-harm

- Previous history of self-harm
- History of mental illness
- Unemployment
- Alcohol- or drug-related problems
- Lack of cooperation with general hospital treatment
- High suicidal intent

(adapted from NICE 2004)

People who self-injure should be offered adequate pain relief, as well as have their wounds treated. They often have quite complex problems, including low self-esteem, eating disorders and substance misuse, and they may find it difficult to engage with professional services. Many people also fall into a repeated pattern of self-injury at times of stress. For these reasons, great care needs to be taken to identify sources of support and to avoid further alienation. Therapeutic work with people who self-harm can include accepting the injuries as part of the person's coping, but aiming to reduce the damage associated with them, *harm reduction*, for example, by providing fresh dressings for the patient to use.

Box 9.5 Care of people who self-harm – summary

- Engage with the patient and manage the episode with a sympathetic approach and clear communication, providing information and offering choices of treatment where these are available
- Provide emergency care, including analgesia where necessary
- Promote safety and reduce harm by advising on the safe management of medications and wounds
- Identify sources of support and effective coping strategies
- Identify risk factors for suicide and repeated acts of self-harm
- Identify physical and mental health problems and support the patient in getting help for these
- Refer on for specialist assessment and management

The longer-term support of people who self-harm is best carried out by mental health specialists, and this will usually involve either a community mental health or liaison psychiatry team. The aims of long-term management are to:

- prevent escalation of self-harm;
- reduce harm arising from self-harm or reduce or stop self-harm;
- reduce or stop other risk-related behaviour;
- improve social or occupational functioning;
- improve quality of life;
- improve any associated mental health conditions.

(NICE 2011b)

Care planning needs to involve the patient and their family and other carers. It should involve a risk management plan, and it should be reviewed at least once a year, and after any episodes of self-harm (NICE 2011b).

Suicide prevention

There were 5,608 suicides in adults in the United Kingdom in 2010 (Office for National Statistics 2011). Suicides rates tend to be fairly consistent over time, and men are far more likely to kill themselves than women: the rate for men in 2010 was 17.0 per 100,000 population and for women 5.3 per 100,000. The rate of suicide is much higher in people who have a history of self-harm, and about a quarter of people who die by suicide attended hospital following an act of self-harm during the previous year (Owens and House 1994). Suicide prevention strategies focus mainly on either primary prevention:

reducing the risks of people turning to self-harm, or secondary prevention: reducing the chances of repetition in people who have self-harmed (Anderson and Jenkins 2006). Given the known risk factors for suicide (Box 9.6), there is the potential for general adult nurses to be involved in both primary and secondary prevention (Box 9.7).

Box 9.6 Suicide risk factors

- Male gender (this includes young men and men over 75 years)
- Mental illness (e.g. depression, schizophrenia)
- Alcohol or drug misuse, particularly when associated with mental health problems
- History of previous self-harm
- Physical illness, particularly long-term conditions including epilepsy, cancer and chronic pain
- Living alone or socially isolated
- Access to lethal means of suicide (e.g. prescription medication, firearms)

(adapted from NICE 2004)

Box 9.7 Suicide prevention strategies for nurses

Primary prevention – reducing the likelihood of self-harm and suicide
- Knowledgeable and sensitive nursing care of common and serious mental illness (e.g. depression, schizophrenia, and alcohol and drug misuse)
- Screening for suicide risk in vulnerable patient groups
- Effective working relationships with mental health teams, including clear lines of referral, to ensure adequate support and treatment for mental illness
- Encouraging greater awareness of mental illness and suicide risk among colleagues and the general population

Secondary prevention – reducing repetition of self-harm and suicide
- Sensitive care in the aftermath of self-harm, engaging patients and reducing alienation
- Identifying those at risk following self-harm and ensuring psychosocial assessment and/or onward referral

---

Reflection point

Within your area of nursing practice, do you encounter people who self-harm or who may be at risk of suicide? What role do you think you and your service would have in helping these people? What are the limits of what you could achieve, and where would you look for support?

Alcohol and drug misuse

Drug misuse refers to the use of any drug in a way that is harmful to the individual. This can include physical and psychological dependence, but it also includes many health and social problems. There is a wide range of drugs that are subject to misuse, some of which are legally available and some that have been made illegal because of the risks associated with their use. However, legality does not represent the level of risk: the most dangerous drug of misuse in the United Kingdom is alcohol, which is legal and freely available.

Alcohol

Alcohol is a very common element of social interaction in many countries of the world, including the United Kingdom. People who drink within the recommended safe levels of intake (Box 9.8) are unlikely to suffer any health problems and may gain health benefits. Drinking to excess, either in binges or as a chronic pattern of drinking over time is, likely to cause health problems, and possibly also social problems (see Box 9.9). Binge drinking is most common in the under 25s, and is associated with an increased risk of alcohol poisoning, accidents, committing acts of violence and being the victim of physical or sexual assault. Chronic drinkers, who tend to be older, often have physical and social problems (see Boxes 9.10 and 9.11) (Strategy Unit 2004).

Box 9.8 Recommended safe levels of alcohol

- Men 3–4 units of alcohol per day, or 21 units a week with alcohol-free days.
- Women 2–3 units of alcohol per day, or 14 units a week with alcohol-free days.
- 1 unit = a small 25 ml measure of spirits (40%) or 125 ml glass of wine (9%)
- 2 units = a pint of ordinary strength beer (4%) or 175 ml glass of wine (12%)
- 3 units = a pint of strong beer or cider (5–5.5%) or 250 ml glass of wine (13%) or 750 ml bottle of alcopops (4%)
- 4 units = 500 ml bottle of strong cider (7.5%)

Box 9.9 Alcohol – key terminology

- *Hazardous drinking*   A pattern of drinking that carries the risk of physical and psychological harm; drinking in excess of the recommended limits.
- *Harmful drinking*   Drinking that is causing physical and psychological harm; drinking 50 units a week in men, and 35 units a week in women.
- *Binge drinking*   Drinking a lot in a short space of time in order to get drunk or feel intoxicated. Also defined as drinking twice the daily recommended limit: in men, 8 units, and in women, 6 units would be a binge.
- *Alcohol dependence*   A syndrome associated with a strong compulsion to drink, difficulty controlling intake, increased tolerance, withdrawal symptoms and increased prioritization of drinking in spite of the problems it causes.

In England, rates of hazardous drinking are estimated at 24 per cent of the population, being twice as common among men, and harmful drinking at 6 per cent for men and 2 per cent for women, with rates of alcohol dependence in the region of 9 per cent for men and 3 per cent for women (McManus et al 2009). Alcohol-related problems contribute to 7 per cent of hospital admissions and up 40 per cent of attendances in emergency departments, and this is higher at peak times (NICE 2011a). In addition to individual health problems, alcohol misuse is responsible for significant social and legal problems (Strategy Unit 2004). Alcohol therefore presents substantial challenges for individuals and their families, for health care services and society as a whole.

Box 9.10 Alcohol – effects on health

- Gastrointestinal: malnutrition, oesophagitis, gastritis, pancreatitis, liver disease
- Neurological: brain and neurological damage, peripheral neuropathy, Wernicke's encephalopathy
- Cardiovascular: arrhythmias, cerebrovascular accidents, hypertension, cardiomyopathy
- Malignancy: head and neck cancers, breast cancer, pancreatic cancer, cancer of the colon
- Reproductive: sexual dysfunction, infertility
- Respiratory: infections, aspiration pneumonia
- Psychological: depression, self-harm and suicidal behaviour
- Other: accidents, acts of violence

Box 9.11 Alcohol – social problems

- Relationship problems
- Domestic violence
- Neglect and abuse of children
- Financial problems: overspending, debt, loss of income
- Loss of days at work and loss of employment
- Homelessness
- Criminal behaviour: theft, violence, sexual assaults, driving offences

---

Responding to the challenge of alcohol misuse

Alcohol misuse is clearly a serious health and social problem. Given the extensive contact that nurses have with those at risk, nurses are well placed to act as a first line of assessment and intervention. Those at risk include people whose health problems could be alcohol related (Box 9.10). Other groups of people who are more likely to have problems with alcohol misuse are the mentally ill, the homeless and roofless sleepers, people who misuse drugs, persistent offenders and young people who have complex multiple needs, for example alcohol and drug misuse, homelessness, mental health problems (Strategy Unit 2004).

There are three primary strategies that nurses can use to aid problem drinkers: screening or assessment (see Box 9.12), brief interventions and referral to specialist services. Identifying alcohol problems early can prevent the development of the serious health problems encountered in chronic drinking. Brief interventions begin by identifying the patient's level of alcohol use and problems associated with this. They are then offered a motivational counselling session that identifies the benefits of cutting down and tips on how to do this, how to set goals for reducing drinking, how to act on this and how to review progress, and it may also involve taking away a self-help booklet (Lock et al 2006). Nurse-led interventions in emergency units (Désy et al 2010), and in general hospital wards (McQueen et al 2011) have resulted in reduced alcohol consumption though it is not clear whether this leads to long-term changes in drinking behaviour.

Box 9.12 Alcohol screening tools

- *Alcohol units* – Asking patients how many units of alcohol they drink in a day and within a week will identify those drinking at hazardous and harmful levels
- *AUDIT* is a 10-item questionnaire that identifies drinking at a hazardous or harmful level by reviewing problems associated with drinking over the past year (Saunders et al 1993)
- *FAST* is 4-item reduced version of AUDIT that is particularly useful for busy settings, accessed at: www.alcohollearningcentre.org.uk/Topics/Browse/BriefAdvice/?parent=4444&child=4570

Alcohol services

There are specialist services for people who misuse alcohol, and it is useful for nurses to familiarize themselves with local services so that they can seek advice and make referrals. These are mostly community based, and involve structured counselling, like motivational interviewing, support for coping on an individual or family basis and community detoxification. Self-help groups such as Alcoholics Anonymous are a source of peer support to people with alcohol problems and their families.

Within either a community or a hospital setting, nurses will encounter patients showing signs of alcohol dependence (Box 9.13) or alcohol withdrawal (Box 9.14). Patients may voluntarily choose to stop drinking and seek help with withdrawal, or they may start withdrawal involuntarily after becoming ill, being admitted to hospital for other treatment or after surgery. Withdrawal can be managed in hospital or in the community. Anyone at risk of delirium tremens or seizures should be offered hospital-based withdrawal, involving the use of benzodiazepines such as chlordiazepoxide or diazepam. Alcohol specialist nurses can have a primary role in supervising hospital-based withdrawal, based on symptom-triggered dosing of benzodiazepines (National Clinical Guideline Centre 2010). Patients who are withdrawing from alcohol can experience acute symptoms of confusion and hallucinations so refer to *Nursing care of psychotic states* and *Nursing care of delirium and dementia* in Chapter 8 for management guidelines.

Box 9.13 Signs of alcohol dependence

- Anxiety and irritability
- Tremor
- Drinking in the morning
- Morning retching
- Amnesia and blackouts
- Withdrawal syndrome and seizures

Box 9.14 Alcohol withdrawal syndrome

Starts six hours after stopping alcohol consumption, and lasts 40–50 hours.

- Anxiety, restlessness
- Tremor
- Sweating
- Nausea, retching
- Tachycardia, hypertension
- Pyrexia
- Hallucinations, both auditory and visual, often disturbing
- Seizures
- Delirium tremens: characterized by confusion, plus the above symptoms, can be severe with circulatory collapse

Box 9.15 Nursing care of people who misuse alcohol – summary

- Be aware of signs of problem drinking
- Screen for alcohol misuse and dependence in people at risk
- Provide health education on alcohol to patients
- Undertake brief motivational interventions where possible
- Refer on for specialist support and withdrawal management where necessary

Case study: alcohol misuse

George Palmer, 22 years old, attended the emergency department in the early hours of a Sunday morning, accompanied by two friends. They had been out drinking and George had fallen after trying to climb up a drainpipe. He had an injury to his ankle that required treatment. He returns to the minor injuries clinic one week later. The clinic nurse, Shirley, takes his history and asks how much he had been drinking on the night of the accident.

He was not sure because he could not remember all of the events of the evening, including the accident. Using a chart with Shirley, they estimate that he had had about 20 units of alcohol during the course of the evening. In an average week he drinks 40 units of alcohol over two or three nights. Shirley provides him with written information about the health implications of drinking, and asks what the consequences of the accident have been for him. He has lost time at work, and will not be able to play football for several weeks, something that is an important part of his life. Shirley asks if he sees benefits to cutting his drinking down, and he agrees he would like to try. They agree what would be a reasonable and safer level of units when he goes out at weekends, and how he could manage this, for example, by skipping rounds of drinks, and explaining to his friends how he wants to keep fit to play football. They agree how he can monitor this and he says he will let Shirley know how he gets on at his next appointment.

Reflection point

- How would you describe George's drinking pattern and level of alcohol use?
- What other forms of assessment could Shirley have used and what additional information could she have learned from this?
- What sorts of problems will George face in cutting down on his drinking?

Drug misuse

There is a wide variety of drugs that are commonly misused, and new drugs are becoming available all of the time; for example, 'legal highs' (see Box 9.16). Well-known illegal drugs include cannabis, cocaine, heroin, crack cocaine, ecstasy and amphetamines. Recreational drug use is fairly common: roughly 10 per cent of adults in England have used illegal drugs within the previous year, and 35 per cent within their lifetime (National Health Information Centre 2007). People who use illegal drugs often also use alcohol and tobacco. Although heroin misuse is relatively rare, it is associated with a high level of health and social problems.

Problem drug use and harm

Within the literature, the term *problem drug use* is common when identifying target populations for intervention. Although it is not well defined, it generally carries a meaning of drug use that is out of control, leads to substantial harm to the user and those around them, and is associated with additional serious social problems. It is also sometimes used to describe the use of heroin and crack cocaine, and often signifies drug dependence (Cave et al 2009). *Drug harm(s)* describes the effects that problem drug use has on the life of the user and those around them, including physical, psychological and social effects (Nutt et al 2010).

Box 9.16 Drugs of misuse

Drug type	Examples	Effects
Cannabis	Marijuana, cannabis resin	Heightened perception, mood changes, relaxation, slowed reaction time, impaired balance, coordination and memory, panic attacks, psychosis
Opioids (these include opiates that are drugs derived from opium, and opioids that are syn-thetic or semi-synthetic)	Opium, heroin, metha-done, buprenorphine	Analgesia, euphoria, psychological numbing, drowsiness, impaired coordination, confusion, slowed breathing
Stimulants	Cocaine, crack cocaine, amphetamine, ecstasy (MDMA)	Euphoria, energy, confidence, hallucinations, tachycardia and hypertension, teeth clenching, tremors, psychosis
Benzodiazepines	Diazepam, lorazepam	Calmness and relaxation, emo-tional clouding, nausea, irritability, aggression, anxiety, depression
Hallucinogens	Lysergic acid diethyl-amide (LSD), mescaline	Mood and perceptual changes (sometimes profound), nausea, anxiety, paranoia, panic
Legal highs	Various – new drugs emerging all the time	Various – e.g. euphoria, energy, mimicking effects of illegal drugs
Dissociative drugs	Ketamine	Feeling separate from your body, impaired motor function, analge-sia, delirium

Some of the most serious health effects of drugs are a result of intravenous drug use, in particular deep vein injecting in areas like the groin. This is most common in users of heroin and crack cocaine. Health problems occurring with intravenous drug use are:

- HIV/AIDS
- hepatitis B and C infection
- collapsed veins, injection-site abscesses
- infections, including septicaemia
- endocarditis
- arthritis and rheumatologic complaints

The lifestyle associated with drug misuse can result in malnutrition, sleep problems, disrupted menstrual cycles and constipation (Neale 2004). It is also associated with accidents, drug overdoses and suicide. There is a strong association between problem drug use and mental health problems, and this can involve drug-induced psychoses and mood disorders.

Problem drug use, including intravenous heroin and crack cocaine use, is also associated with substantial social problems. These include problems with family members, neglect of children, employment and financial problems, and criminal behaviour, and there is a considerable overlap with alcohol-related social problems (Box 9.11). Homelessness is very common among problem drug users; at approximately 25 per cent, it is seven times more common than among the general population, though least common where family support is maintained (Kemp et al 2006).

Some drugs lead to more harm than others. A complex analysis of the harm caused by different drugs across different physical, psychological and social criteria, and divided into harm to user and harm to others, found that three drugs in particular are associated with most harm. These are alcohol, heroin and crack cocaine. In terms of harm to the user, the order was crack cocaine, heroin, then alcohol, and in terms of harm to others, alcohol was by far the most harmful, followed by heroin then crack cocaine (Nutt et al 2010).

Problem drug use – assessment

Patients with problem drug use should be assessed thoroughly to identify their current state of health and any other problems that would benefit from professional intervention. It is often helpful to involve a social worker in the assessment process, especially if the patient has dependent children. One of the aims of assessment is to identify patients who are at risk. A thorough assessment will include drug use, health, criminal involvement and social functioning (Box 9.17). This will provide the basis for either a brief intervention or onward referral to specialist services. It is also important to be aware of the signs and symptoms of drug withdrawal. Box 9.18 gives the signs of opioid withdrawal but many of these, for example irritability and restlessness, also occur with other drugs.

Box 9.17 Psychosocial assessment of problem drug use

Drug and alcohol use
- Which drugs are used, including alcohol and tobacco, and in what amounts
- Pattern, frequency and which route is used to take drugs
- Symptoms of dependence
- Source of drugs, including prescribed medication

Physical and psychological health
- Physical problems, including complications of drugs and alcohol use
- Blood-borne infections, risk behaviours and sexual health, including pregnancy

- Psychological problems, including depression, anxiety and serious mental illness, and contact with mental health services
- History of self-harm, abuse or trauma

Criminal involvement and offending
- Any outstanding legal issues, including arrests, fines and warrants
- Involvement with workers in the criminal justice system (e.g. probation)

Social functioning
- Current social circumstances, including family, partner
- Housing, employment, benefits and financial problems
- Childcare issues, including parenting, pregnancy and child protection

(DoH 2007)

Box 9.18 Signs of opioid withdrawal

- Anxiety, restlessness and irritability
- Yawning, coughing, sneezing, runny nose
- Tachycardia, hypertension
- Dilated pupils
- Cool, clammy skin
- Nausea, diarrhoea
- Tremor
- Abdominal cramps
- Craving

Drug misuse – strategies for management

In any health care situation, where drug misuse is identified, nurses can carry out a brief intervention, similar to those for people who misuse alcohol: provide information, health education, motivational counselling and explore options for professional support or self-help groups (Compton et al 1999). If alcohol or tobacco is used, support can also be given to reduce or stop its use. People who misuse drugs often feel that they are not understood or that they are treated in a judgemental fashion by hospital staff (Neale et al 2008). Engagement and a non-judgemental attitude are therefore important aspects of nursing care.

Specialist services for people who misuse opioid drugs can be based on strategies of reduction of drug use, harm reduction or abstinence from drugs:

- *Pharmacological management* of opioid misuse. Safer, non-injected opioids like methadone or buprenorphine can be given on prescription at pharmacies.

- *Harm reduction*, including advice on safe preparation and injection practices, needle exchange and avoiding overdosing.
- *Contingency management*, which involves goal-setting with financial incentives for achieving those goals. Goals can include reduction of drug use, safer use of or abstinence from drugs.

Psychotherapy is sometimes offered to people who misuse drugs, including cannabis or amphetamines. Approaches used include cognitive behavioural therapy (CBT), motivational interviewing, group or couple therapy and psychodynamic therapies (NICE 2007).

Nursing care of people with problem drug use – summary

- Engage people who misuse drugs and work with them in a non-judgemental way
- Be aware of signs of drug misuse and dependence
- Provide health education on drug misuse to patients
- Undertake brief motivational interventions where possible
- Liaise with specialist drug services and general psychiatric services

References

Anderson, M. and Jenkins, R. (2006) The national suicide prevention strategy for England: the reality of a national strategy for the nursing profession, *Journal of Psychiatric and Mental Health Nursing*, 13, 641–650.

Cave, J., Hunt, P., Ismail, S., Levitt, R., Liccardo Piccula, R., Rabinovich, L., Rubin, J. and Weed, K. (2009) *Tackling Problem Drug Use*. London: National Audit Office.

Commons Treloar, A. and Lewis, A. (2008) Professional attitudes towards deliberate self-harm in patients with borderline personality disorder, *Australian and New Zealand Journal of Psychiatry*, 42, 578–584.

Compton, P., Monahan, G. and Simmons-Cody, H. (1999) Motivational interviewing: an effective brief intervention for alcohol and drug abuse patients, *Nurse Practitioner*, 24 (11), 27–49.

Department of Health (England) and the devolved administrations (DoH) (2007) *Drug Misuse and Dependence: UK Guidelines on Clinical Management*. London: Department of Health (England), the Scottish Government, Welsh Assembly Government and Northern Ireland Executive.

Désy, P., Kunz Howard, P., Perhats, C. and Li, S. (2010) Alcohol screening, brief intervention, and referral to treatment conducted by emergency nurses: an impact evaluation, *Journal of Emergency Nursing*, 36 (6), 538–545.

Dettmore, D., Kolanowski, A. and Boustani, M. (2009) Aggression in persons with dementia: use of nursing theory to guide clinical practice, *Geriatric Nursing*, 30 (1), 8–17.

Ewing, J. (1984) Detecting alcoholism: the CAGE questionnaire, *Journal of the American Medical Association* (JAMA), 252 (14), 1905–1907.

Hahn, S., Müller, M., Needham, I., Dassen, T., Kok, G. and Halfens, R. (2010) Factors associated with patient and visitor violence experienced by nurses in general hospitals in Switzerland: a cross-sectional study, *Journal of Clinical Nursing*, 19, 3535–3546.

Hjelmeland, H., Hawton, Nordvik, H., Bille-Brahe, U., de Leo, D., Fekete, S., Grad, O., Haring, C., Kerkhof, J., Lönnqvist, J., Michel, K., Salander Renberg, E., Schmidtke, A., van Heeringen, K. and Wassermann, D. (2002) Why people engage in parasuicide: a cross-cultural study of intentions, *Suicide and Life-threatening Behaviour*, 32 (4), 295–303.

Horrocks, J., Price, S., House, A. and Owens, D (2003) Self-injury attendances in the accident and emergency department: clinical database study, *British Journal of Psychiatry*, 183, 34–39.

Johnson, M. and Webb, C. (1995) Rediscovering unpopular patients: the concept of social judgement, *Journal of Advanced Nursing*, 21, 466–475.

Kemp, P., Neale, J. and Robertson, M. (2006) Homelessness among problem drug users: prevalence, risk factors and trigger events, *Health and Social Care in the Community*, 14 (4), 319–328.

Lock, C., Kaner, E., Heather, N., Doughty, J., Crawshaw, A., McNamee, P., Purdy, S. and Pearson, P. (2006) Effectiveness of nurse-led brief alcohol intervention: a cluster randomized controlled trial, *Journal of Advanced Nursing*, 54 (4), 426–439.

Luck, L., Jackson, D. and Usher, K. (2007) STAMP: components of observable behaviour that indicate potential for violence in emergency departments, *Journal of Advanced Nursing*, 59 (1), 11–19.

McAllister, M., Creedy, D., Moyle, W. and Farrugia, C. (2002) Nurses' attitudes towards clients who self-harm, *Journal of Advanced Nursing*, 40 (5), 578–586.

McManus, S., Meltzer, H., Brugha, T., Bebbington, P. and Jenkins, R. (2009) Adult psychiatric morbidity in England, 2007: results of a household survey, NHS Information Centre for Health and Social Care, Leeds.

McQueen, J., Howe, T., Allan, L. and Mains, D. (2011) Brief interventions for heavy alcohol users admitted to general hospital wards, *The Cochrane Library*. Available online at www. mrw.interscience.wiley.com/cochrane/clsysrev/articles/CD005191/pdf_fs.html

National Clinical Guideline Centre (2010) *Alcohol Use Disorders: Diagnosis and Clinical Management of Alcohol-related Physical Complications*, Clinical Guideline 100. London: National Clinical Guideline Centre. Available online at www.guidance.nice.org.uk/CG100

National Health Information Centre (2007) *Statistics on Drug Misuse: England, 2007*. London: The Information Centre, Lifestyles Statistics. Available online at www.ic.nhs.uk/pubs/drugmisuse07

National Institute for Clinical Excellence (NICE) (2004) *Self-harm. The Short-term Physical and Psychological Management and Secondary Prevention of Self-harm in Primary and Secondary Care*, National Clinical Practice Guideline 16. London: NICE. Available online at www.publications.nice.org.uk/self-harm-cg16

National Institute for Clinical Excellence (NICE) (2007) *Drug Misuse: Psychosocial Interventions*, NICE Clinical Guideline 51. London: NICE. Available online at www.guidance.nice.org.uk/CG51

National Institute for Clinical Excellence (NICE) (2011a) *Alcohol-Use Disorders: Diagnosis, Assessment and Management of Harmful Drinking and Alcohol Dependence*, National Clinical Practice Guideline 115. London: NICE. Available online at www.guidance.nice.org.uk/CG115/Guidance

National Institute for Clinical Excellence (NICE) (2011b) *Self-harm: Longer-term management*, National Clinical Practice Guideline 133. London: NICE. Available online at www.guidance.nice.org.uk/cg133/

Neale, J. (2004) Measuring the health of Scottish drug users, *Health and Social Care in the Community*, 12 (3), 202–211.

Neale, J., Tompkins, C. and Sheard, L. (2008) Barriers to accessing generic health and social care services: a qualitative study of injecting drug users, *Health and Social Care in the Community*, 16 (2), 147–154.

Needham, I., Abderhalden, C., Halfens, R., Fischer, J. and Dassen, T. (2005) Non-somatic effects of patient aggression on nurses: a systematic review, *Journal of Advanced Nursing*, 49 (3), 283–296.

Nutt, D., King, L. and Phillips, L. (2010) Drug harms in the UK: a multicriteria decision analysis, *The Lancet*, 376 (9752), 1558–1565.

O'Connell, B., Young, J., Brooks, J., Hutchings, J. and Lofthouse, J. (2000) Nurses' perceptions of the nature and frequency of aggression in general ward settings and high dependency areas, *Journal of Clinical Nursing*, 9, 602–610.

Office for National Statistics (2011) *Suicide Rates in the United Kingdom, 2006 to 2010*. London: Office for National Statistics. Available online at www.ons.gov.uk/ons/dcp171778_254113.pdf

Owens, D. and House, A. (1994) General hospital services for deliberate self-harm, *Journal of the Royal College of Physicians*, 28 (1), 370–371.

Regel, S. (2002) Staff support in trauma and critical care settings, in Regel, S. and Roberts, D. (eds) *Mental Health Liaison: A Handbook for Nurse and Health Professionals*, pp. 309–326.

Roberts, D. and Mackay, G. (1999) A nursing model of overdose assessment, *Nursing Times*, 95 (3), 58–60.

Saunders, J., Aasland, O., Babor, T., de la Fuente, J. and Grant, M. (1993) Development of the Alcohol Use Disorders Identification Test (AUDIT): WHO collaborative project on early detection of persons with harmful alcohol consumption – II, *Addiction*, 88, 791–804.

Shattell, M. (2004) Nurse–patient interaction: a review of the literature, *Journal of Clinical Nursing*, 13 (6), 714–722.

Stockwell, F. (1972) *The Unpopular Patient*. London: Royal College of Nursing and National Council of Nurses of the United Kingdom. Available online at www.rcn.org.uk/__data/assets/pdf_file/0005/235508/series_1_number_2.pdf

Stokes, G. (2000) *Challenging Behaviour in Dementia: A Person-Centred Approach*. Milton Keynes: Speechmark.

Strategy Unit (2004) *Alcohol Harm Reduction Project*. London: Cabinet Office. Available online at www.erpho.org.uk/viewResource.aspx?id=14668

Svirko, E. and Hawton, K. (2007) Self-injurious behaviour and eating disorders: the extent and nature of the problem, *Suicide and Life-Threatening Behavior*, 37 (4), 409–421.

Taylor, T., Hawton, K., Fortune, S. and Kapur, N. (2009) Attitudes towards clinical services among people who self-harm: systematic review, *British Journal of Psychiatry*, 194, 104–110.

Further reading

Reece, J. (2005) The language of cutting: initial reflections on a study of the experiences of self-injury in a group of women and nurses, *Issues in Mental Health Nursing*, 26, 561–574.

Stokes, G. (2000) *Challenging Behaviour in Dementia. A Person-Centred Approach*. Milton Keynes: Speechmark.

Alcohol Learning Centre: www.alcohollearningcentre.org.uk/

MIND Guide to Understanding Self-harm: www.mind.org.uk/help/diagnoses_and_conditions/self-harm?gclid=CLKyvcO6o7ECFYUKfAodjxhzjQ

Index